Innovative Approaches for Conservation and Improvement of Indigenous Bovine Genetic Resources

Innovative Approaches for Conservation and Improvement of Indigenous Bovine Genetic Resources

Dr K.P. Ramesha
Principal Scientist & Head of the Station
Animal Genetics & Breeding, Southern Regional Station
ICAR-National Dairy Research Institute, Bengaluru

Dr Mukund A. Kataktalware
Senior Scientist
Livestock Production Management, Southern Regional Station,
ICAR- National Dairy Research Institute, Bengaluru

Dr S. Jeyakumar
Principal Scientist
Animal Reproduction & Gynaecology, Southern Regional Station
ICAR-National Dairy Research Institute, Bengaluru

Dr D.N. Das
Principal Scientist
Animal Genetics & Breeding, Southern Regional Station
ICAR-National Dairy Research Institute, Bengaluru

Dr A. Kumaresan
Principal Scientist
Animal Reproduction & Gynaecology, Southern Regional Station
ICAR-National Dairy Research Institute, Bengaluru

International Books & Periodical Supply Service

(Publisher of Scientific Books)

38, NISHANT KUNJ, PITAM PURA MAIN ROAD
DELHI-110034 (India)
Phone : 011-27352078, Mobile : 09810146811, E-mail : hkjain1975@yahoo.com

Published by :

International Books & Periodical Supply Service

(Publisher of Scientific Books)
38, NISHANT KUNJ, PITAM PURA MAIN ROAD
DELHI-110034 (India)
Phone : 011-27352078, Mobile : 09810146811, E-mail : hkjain1975@yahoo.com

ISBN 978-93-88892-05-6

Composed, Designed & Printed in India

About the Editors

Dr K.P. Ramesha is heading Southern Regional Station of ICAR-NDRI, Bengaluru. He earned B.V.Sc. and M.V.Sc. degrees from Veterinary College, Bangalore and obtained Ph.D. from NDRI, Karnal in 1991. He earned PG Diploma in IPR and Master of IP Law. He did pioneering work in the area of male fertility assessment, livestock genomics, embryo biotechnology, improvement of indigenous cattle, transcriptomics, and screening of males for genetic diseases & cytogenetic abnormalities and proteomics of milk and IPR issues. He has successfully completed 22 research projects including DBT, NATP, Karnataka Government and NDDB funded projects and guided 10 PG and 6 Ph.D. Scholars. Due to his efforts Malnad Gidda- dwarf cattle of Karnataka has been registered as a recognized breed. He has been empanelled as Scientific Advisor under Patent Act. He has published more than 95 research articles, about 100 scientific and technical publications. He has edited and published several books, book chapters and monographs. He has 3 patent applications to his credit. Dr Ramesha is the recipient of many awards including Fakrudhin Ali Ahmed Award for the biennium 2004-2005 by ICAR, New Delhi, Dr G.B. Singh Memorial Award, 1993 of the Indian Society for Study of Animal Reproduction, Visiting fellow of JNCASR, Bangalore, Indira Gandhi Sadbhavana Gold Medal Award, 2013 by Global Economic Progress and Research Association, Best Veterinarian Award, 2011-13 by Karnataka Veterinary Association, Best Zoologist Award, 2013 by Society for Applied Biotechnology. He has been elected as a Fellow of Society for Association for the Advancement of Biodiversity Science during 2013. Justice Sri. M.N. Venkatachaliah, the Former Chief Justice of India conferred Sir J.C. Bose Memorial Award from Indian Science Monitor, (Regd.), Chennai to Dr Ramesha on 18th January, 2015. He is the Fellow of Indian Dairy Association, India; Fellow of National Academy of Veterinary Sciences (India) and National Academy of Dairy Science (India).

Dr Mukund A. Kataktalware is presently working as a Senior Scientist (Livestock Production Management), Southern Regional Station of ICAR-NDRI, Bengaluru. He obtained B.V.Sc. & A.H. from Nagpur Veterinary College, Nagpur in 1998 and PG (LPM) in 2000 & Ph.D. (LPM) in 2004 from ICAR-NDRI, Karnal. He joined the ARS in 2004 at ICAR-NRC on Yak, Dirang, Arunachal Pradesh and since 2009 working at SRS, ICAR-NDRI, Bengaluru. He earned PG Diploma in IPR from IGNOU, New Delhi in 2012. He has successfully completed 25 research projects (Seven as Principal Investigator and 18 as Co-PI) including seven externally funded projects viz., ICAR Network Project 'Adaptation and facilitation of livestock to impending climatic changes through shelter management', ICAR sponsored 'National Innovations on Climate Resilient Agriculture', Karnataka Livestock Development Agency sponsored 'Evaluation and Improvement of Indigenous Cattle of Malnad Region of Karnataka', etc. Presently, he is associated with ICAR sponsored project 'Farmer FIRST', Karnataka Biodiversity Board sponsored 'Documentation of Traditional Knowledge of Livestock Keepers of Karnataka State' and MoEFCC-KLDA sponsored 'Proteo-Genomic approach to elucidate productive and reproductive performance of Malnad Gidda, Deoni and Hallikar breeds of cattle' projects. He has guided six PG Scholars. He was also involved in cryopreservation of yak semen, registration of Malnad Gidda breed and cryopreservation of Malnad Gidda semen. He has published about 65 research papers, three books, 20 book chapters, five technical bulletins, 40 technical articles, and three review articles. His present research interest includes cryopreservation and improvement of bovine semen quality, climate change, lameness, quality milk production, etc.

Dr S. Jeyakumar was born on 1st June, 1972 at T. Kalluppatti, Madurai District of Tamil Nadu and graduated from Madras Veterinary College. He completed his Master's and Doctoral degree in Animal Reproduction from IVRI and TANUVAS, respectively. He joined ARS in the year 2000. His major research interest is in dairy animal reproduction particularly in the field of controlled breeding, ET and ultrasound-guided ovum pick-up and *in-vitro* embryo production. During his long service in Andman and Nicobar Islands, he carried out research on genetic up-gradation of local cattle and buffalo for improved production. A hybrid goat "Boer cross goat" was developed and propagated using A.I. technology. He has pioneered in the development of modified ultrasonography method to study/diagnose physiopathological changes in the teat, udder of crossbred cows, testis in goat and avian reproductive ultrasonography. He has significantly contributed in the area of breed characterization, evaluation, documentation, conservation of livestock biodiversity and especially he was responsible for registration of two new breeds viz. Nicobari Pig and Teressa Goat by ICAR. He has completed 9 external and institute funded projects as PI and contributed to about 30 projects as co-investigator. Involved in teaching and guided as a mentor under Women Scientist Scheme (DST), 2 M.V.Sc., dissertation, 5 M.Sc. and 2 summer training dissertations. He has published about 100 research papers in national and international journals and 120 research abstracts. He has published 5 books, written 5 books chapters, 10 popular/technical articles, 10 manuals/teaching aids, 8 technical folders, 6 extensions/ technical bulletins and 1 policy document. He is a recipient of 25 awards/ certificate of recognition, notably 2 Young Scientist Award and Merit of

Excellence award, 10 best paper/poster awards, an Associateship and a Fellow award from recognized academy/societies.

Dr D.N. Das has research experience of 23 years in the areas of Cytogenetics, Animal Breeding, Molecular Genetics and Transcriptomics. He has contributed for 7 years towards yak genetic improvement. Presently focused in areas bovine genetic resources for characterization, evaluation and genetic improvement of indigenous cattle with special reference to Deoni breed towards improvement of disease tolerance, adaptability and lactation performances. Published 85 research papers of International and National repute. He has guided 8 Ph.D. and 7 M.V.Sc. students. He has handled 8 externally funded research projects including two inter-institute collaborative projects. Presently, he is working in the area of controlling early embryonic mortality in buffaloes using CRISPR/ Cas9 tool.

Dr A. Kumaresan is presently working as a Principal Scientist (Animal Reproduction and Gynaecology) at Southern Regional Station of ICAR-National Dairy Research Institute, Bengaluru. Previously he worked as a Senior Scientist at ICAR-NDRI, Karnal and as a Scientist at ICAR Research Complex for NEH Region. He completed B.V.Sc. from Madras Veterinary College (TANUVAS) and M.V.Sc. and Ph.D. from Indian Veterinary Research Institute, Bareilly. He is a recipient of BOYSCAST Fellowship from the Department of Science and Technology and carried out post-Doc at Swedish Agricultural University (Sweden). He also participated in the JICA training program at Singosari (Indonesia) and awarded as best participant among 14 countries. He has successfully completed 18 externally funded and in-house research projects. His research and teaching contribution have been recognized by ICAR by awarding prestigious National awards viz. Lal Bahadur Shastri Outstanding Young Scientist Award (two times - in 2007 and 2015), Fakhruddin Ali Ahmed Award for Outstanding Research in Tribal Farming Systems (2010) and Bharat Ratna Dr C. Subramaniam Outstanding Teacher Award (2017). He is also honoured with best teacher award and Dr S. K. Sirohi Memorial Outstanding Researcher Award by ICAR-NDRI, Karnal. He authored 14 books, 10 bulletins, 24 book chapters including one chapter in Handbook of Animal Husbandry (ICAR), 34 technical articles, several extension folders and published 182 research papers in journals of International and National repute. He guided 14 M.V.Sc. and 13 Ph.D. scholars as Major Advisor. He is the fellow of National Academy of Dairy Sciences and Indian Society for Study of Animal Reproduction and an Associate of National Academy of Agricultural Sciences.

Preface

Dairying is an important sub-sector of Indian agriculture and milk group has the highest contribution to livestock sector output. India is a mega biodiversity hub of animal genetic resources (AnGR) with 184 indigenous breeds of livestock and poultry with unique traits, which include 43 for cattle, 16 for buffaloes, 34 for goats, 43 for sheep, 7 for horses & ponies, 9 for camels, 8 for pigs, 2 for donkeys, 1 for yaks, 19 for chicken, 1 for ducks and 1 for geese. Besides recognised breeds, there are populations of livestock and poultry in various geographical locations with unique traits. Indigenous livestock has evolved over a long time in the diverse, stressful, tropical environment with adaptive traits. This situation enables them to live and endanger in these conditions. The milk productivity of indigenous cow, crossbred cow, buffalo and goat is only 3.41, 7.33, 5.76 and 0.45 kg/day in the year 2015-16, respectively which needs to be improved substantially. Conservation of indigenous animal genetic resources has attained greater importance against the backdrop of climate change scenario. At the international level, Convention on Biological Diversity (CBD) of United Nations and Trade-Related Aspects of Intellectual Property (TRIPs) Agreement of World Trade Organization are the two major agreements governing access and rights over genetic resources. As India is a signatory to CBD and TRIPs Agreement and also, ratified Global Plan of Action on Animal Genetic Resources, it is obligatory for India to develop suitable legislation to protect and improve livestock biodiversity and associated traditional knowledge.

The foremost pre-requisite for climate resilient livestock production system is maintaining animal breeds, which are well-adapted to local geo-climatic conditions, feed resources, parasites, and known to have a high tolerance to endemic diseases. Therefore, conservation and improvement of indigenous animal genetic resources have attained greater importance against the backdrop of climate change scenario, particularly in the IPR era. It is absolutely necessary to make concerted efforts for applying modern technologies for the conservation of indigenous germplasm and identification and protection of those traits, which are sure but against the adversities of climate change.

We are grateful to Dr R.R.B. Singh, Acting Director, ICAR-NDRI, Karnal for his valuable guidance and inputs in the preparation of this publication. We also take this opportunity to thank all the authors for enriching this publication with their valuable inputs. We are hopeful that this book will be useful to the students, teachers and scientists, who are devoted to the conservation and improvement of indigenous bovine genetic resources.

February 18, 2019 **Editors**

Contents

Chapter 1

Bovine Genetic Resources: Status and Strategies for Productivity Enhancement through Emerging Technologies in the Climate Change Scenario

K.P. Ramesha, N. Azaharuddin and A. Kumaresan

India has rich and diverse genetic resources of livestock and poultry in the form of a large number of species, breeds, and strains within a species. India is home to 184 indigenous breeds of livestock and poultry with unique traits, which include 43 for cattles, 16 for buffaloes, 34 for goats, 43 for sheeps, 7 for horses & ponies, 9 for camels, 8 for pigs, 2 for donkeys, 1 for yak, 19 for chicken, 1 for duck and 1 for geese. Besides recognized breeds, there are populations of livestock and poultry in various geographical locations with unique traits. Cattle and buffaloes rearing has been an integral part of the socio-economic and cultural fabric of rural India since time immemorial. As per the Basic Animal Husbandry Statistics (BAHS) 2012, in India there are about 56.7 per cent of world's buffaloes (105.05 million) with 1st position, 12.5 per cent cattle (199.07 million) with 2nd position, 20.4 per cent small ruminants comprising 144 million goats and 72 million sheep with 2nd and 3rd position, respectively in the world. The Indian breeds of livestock are suited to tropical climatic conditions, are able to resist the heat stress, need less water, can walk long distances, survive on local grasses and resist tropical diseases. They can also be turned into high producers given the right kind of feed and the environment. Indigenous livestock generally requires low maintenance energy. Thus, the impact of climate change will be minimal on low and medium producing animals as compared to high yielding animals.

Bovine milk has fat, carbohydrates, minerals, vitamins, and anti-microbial substances and other health-promoting agents. Casein makes upto about 80% of the protein in the milk. Beta casein is made up of 209 amino acids linked together in sequence. Milk from Indian zebu cattle and buffaloes contain only A2 allele of beta-casein protein, which is considered to be safe for human consumption, whereas A1 allele of beta casein is found to have higher frequency in most of *B. taurus* breeds, which has been implicated in certain diseases, viz. type 1 Diabetes Mellitus, ischemic heart disease, arteriosclerosis and neurological disorders, such as autism and schizophrenia. The difference in A1 and A2 beta-casein is the amino acid histidine in A_1 and proline in A_2 at position 67. The indigenous cow's milk has a high level of Conjugated Linoleic Acid (CLA) content (a vital health promoter) besides a rich source of carotenoids, Vit. D and Vit. B_{12} besides anti-microbial substances viz. lactoferrin, lysozyme, and immunoglobulins. The content of lactoferrin, well-known anti-microbial and anti-viral substance is higher in desi cow milk as compared to crossbred and buffalo milk. Lactoferrin also inhibits fungal and parasitic infections.

India has only 2.4 per cent world's area, 7.3 per cent of the global arable land and 4.2 per cent of the world's water. India is home to 17 and 11 per cent of global human and livestock population. Driven by the structural changes in the agricultural sector and food consumption patterns in the last few decades, the utility of livestock has undergone a transformation with their importance, as a source of quality food has increased. The greatest challenge of the millennium is to produce quality food by increasing production and productivity of agricultural commodities manifolds to meet the requirements of an exponentially growing population with the same/reduced resource base of land and water. These sectors are evolving in response to surging demand for food due to population growth, sustained income and economic growth, urbanization, burgeoning middle-income class and changing lifestyles. The task becomes even more onerous set against climate change and limited natural resources and their constraints (water and soil footprint) and reducing cultivable land. The need is to develop technologies that improve productivity and enable farmers to produce more with fewer resources, reducing the impact on the environment.

The assemblage of the breeds and populations having traits and unique characters is a source of food, fiber and a host of other services, and this assemblage is phrased as Animal Genetic Resource (AnGR). The term AnGR encompasses the genetic material of animals, covering semen, egg and live animals, DNA molecules, RNA, proteins and other microphysical genetic material (Tvedt *et al.*, 2007). It is very essential to maintain genetic diversity to respond to situations like climate change and emerging diseases and to adapt to production systems. Over the centuries, indigenous livestock breeds have adapted to local conditions. Darwinian adaptations of indigenous cattle in relation to their ability to tolerate heat and parasites as well as their ability to survive and produce milk and capacity to work in harsh conditions under poor quality feed and fodder is yet to be fully understood and exploited for further improvements. The main objectives of the Indian National Plan of Action for AnGR are to ensure a strategic and comprehensive approach in achieving the sustainable use, development, and conservation of animal genetic resources, to increase and improve food production and food security, alleviate poverty and contribute to rural development and its role in society for cultural values. At the international level Global plan of action for AnGR, the first internationally agreed framework halt the erosion of livestock diversity and support the sustainable use, development and conservation of AnGR was adopted by delegates from 109 countries at the International Technical Conference on Animal Genetic Resources for Food and Agriculture, 3-7 Sept., 2007, in Interlaken, Switzerland.

India has some of the best breeds of cattle with traits for dairy, drought power, and dual purposes and best breeds of buffaloes. These breeds are essentially the products of long-term natural selection and are better adapted to tropical fodder, environment, and diseases, and perform under low and medium inputs in different ecological niches. Thus, indigenous breeds are well-adapted to the harsh climate, resistant to common tropical diseases and can subsist on poor quality crop residual roughages, grasses, and scanty drinking water. Indigenous cows also could be turned into high milk producers, given the right kind of feed and environment. Under the prevailing conditions, it is not possible to change the production system to suit them and mimic the systems used in developed countries. The grain-based livestock farming has led to the diverting of valuable food crops away from human consumption.

Indian Dairy Sector

Dairying is an important sub-sector of Indian agriculture and milk group has the highest contribution to livestock sector output (68.22%). About 70% of milk is produced by marginal and small farmers, owning

2-4 animals. The different production systems like zero input-low output, low input-moderate output, intensive input-high output are characteristics of the dairy production system in India (Ramesha and Divya, 2013). Dairy sector has shown a constant and sustainable growth despite limited investment from public and the private sector. A perusal of the Fig.1 clearly shows that the production of milk in India has increased substantially over the years. The annual growth rate in milk production during the year 2015-16 was 6.28% while the average growth rate in milk production in the world is around 1.5%. However, a paradigm shift is required in the dairy sector from a production orientation to quality and cost orientation in the WTO era (Ramesha and Jayaraj Rao, 2013).

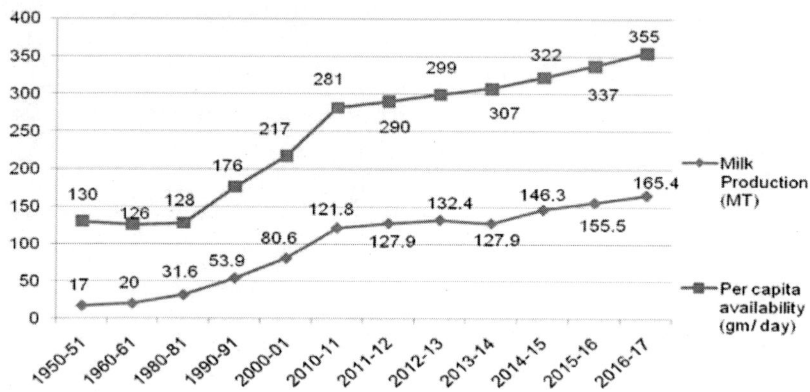

Figure 1*:* Milk production dynamics in India; Source*:* Annual Report (2017-18), DAHD & F, Govt. of India

Dairy animals in India are reared with multiple objectives, besides providing milk also provide a diverse range of output for agriculture, irrigation, manure, and transport; fibre and leather goods and their rearing systems are different from developed countries. The drought-prone semi-arid regions are characterized by a major animal component, as animals can exploit resources that cannot support intensive crop cultivation on a sustainable basis. Cross-breeding of indigenous cattle with exotic high yielding breeds started in the 1960s and currently, the contribution of crossbred cattle to total milk production is around 24 per cent. The adaptation of temperate exotic breeds or their crossbreds out of crossing with Indian breeds needs sophisticated and scientific management to exploit their full production potential under the tropical climate of India. Yet another important problem is the disposal of crossbred males, as farmers don't prefer them for the draft purpose. Even now, about 53 % of milk production in India comes from buffaloes. The milk productivity of indigenous cow, crossbred cow, buffalo, and goat is only 3.41, 7.33, 5.76 and 0.45 kg/day in the year 2015-16, respectively. The differences in milk production of crossbreds and indigenous milch breeds do not seem to be substantial, considering the fact that not much selection has gone into the improvement of indigenous breeds for milk yield. India is the largest milk producer with 160.35 mt (18.5% of the total world milk production) during 2015-16 from 298 million cattle and buffaloes, which is 17.54% of the total world bovine population. In contrast, USA and New Zealand are producing 11.7 and 2.7% of milk from 9.47 and 1.1% of the total world bovine population. Average milk production/cow/year in developed countries viz. USA, Sweden, Denmark is above 7500 kg while in India is only 1200 kg, which clearly indicates the need for productivity enhancement in them.

Recently, several measures have been initiated by the Government of India to increase the productivity of milch animals. Among Indigenous breeds, cows producing good quality milk in lactation have been recorded under Central Herd Registration Scheme for breeds like Gir (3038-3263 kg), Ongole (2000-2544 kg) and Haryana (1671-4015 kg). Even among Maland Gidda-dwarf cattle with a body weight of 80-120 kgs, many cows give 3-4 kgs of milk per day with regular calving under low input production system (Ramesha, 2013). This indicates that there exists the genetic potential for high milk production in indigenous breeds.

Indian Breeds Abroad

India has contributed richly to the international livestock gene pool and improvement of animal production in the world. Brahman cattle are found in 45 countries while the Sahiwal breed is found in 29 countries (Ramesha *et al.*, 2007 and Ramesha *et al.*, 2008). Many cattle breeds of Indian origin have made a major contribution to the development of composite breeds elsewhere in the world. The world's best Gir cows, today, give 5500 litres of milk on an average per lactation of 307 days (Sharma, 2011). In recent years, Brazil has emerged as the world's biggest supplier of improved cattle embryos and semen of Indian origin. The demand for Indian breeds is particularly high from the African and South-east Asian countries. As these breeds are suitable for tropical conditions, these countries find improved cattle germplasm to be ideal for their cattle breeding programmes (Sharma, 2011).

Special characters of Indigenous cattle

Indigenous breeds are well-known for heat tolerance, hardiness and ability to survive and perform even under stressful conditions and low input regimes. Zebu cattle have the ability to convert low protein, high fibre roughage materials into high-grade foodstuffs with the aid of omasal symbionts. They have the ability to reverse down metabolism during extremes of scarcity but show a quick response in the form of better reproductive and productive efficiency, when nutrients are plentiful. Zebu cattle are efficient foragers and their tight sheath and small teats avoid injuries during grazing. The sloppy rumps in draft breeds make them suitable for quick and hard work. The white or light coloured, short, sleek, densely, reflecting and glistering coat in indigenous cattle does not attract vectors and dislodge them. Flexible tail tip helps as a brush to repel vectors. Premunity is high and reticuloendothelial system is well-developed in zebu cattle. Usually, longevity is more than 15 years with high reproduction rates and more number of lifetime calves and many animals give more than 15 calves in their lifetime. They have outstanding mothering ability. They calve with ease and dystokia is rarely reported. There is a great degree of genetic variation in indigenous breeds of livestock with respect to their size, productivity, growth rate, reproductive efficiency, which can be made use for the improvement of livestock worldwide.

Indigenous cattle have a lower basal metabolic rate, better capacity for heat dissipation through cutaneous evaporation and thus, adaptation to tropical heat and resistance to diseases, especially the tick-borne diseases than taurine cattle. Indigenous cattle possess natural resistance to various insects, as their skin has a dense texture, making it difficult for blood-sucking insects to penetrate. Several studies indicate the differential disease resistance of indigenous cattle compared to exotic cattle on *Theileria parva* (Ndungu *et al.*, 2005), on tick infestation (Mwangi *et al.*, 1998), on symptoms of babesiosis (Aulakh *et al.*, 2005). The CRC (2006) work in Australia confirms tick resistance but also shows the poorer temperament in Brahman cattle. Most of the indigenous cattle can withstand and graze even at atmospheric temperatures of 40°C. Aggarwal and Singh (2006) reported Upper (UCT) and Lower Critical Temperatures (LCT) for different breed types as 38°C and 10°C, respectively for Indigenous breeds, 24°C and 2°C for Jersey and crosses, 20°C and 10°C, respectively for Holsteins. Ghosh *et al.* (2006) report temperatures at which milk production starts to reduce as 21°C for Holsteins,

24/27°C for Jersey and Brown Swiss and 32°C for Zebu type. Due to these special characteristics of indigenous cattle, they are able to conceive after drought while crossbreds fail to conceive after lack of feed and water, and many times sent to the slaughter house (Ramesha, 2003). The study conducted in Kerala Veterinary University showed that Vechur cattle did not show symptoms of heat stress even after exposure to sunlight. There had been an only a slight increase in body temperature after exposure to the sun (Venkatachalapathy and Iype, 2010). The extensive area covered by the dewlap, loose body skin, more sweat glands, and hair coat play a vital role in its heat tolerance.

Impact of climate change on Bovine Genetic Resources

Potential impacts of climate change on bovine production in India are yet to be exhaustively studied. The temperature increase in mid-altitude and in high altitude is liable to amend pasture production by incrementing the season of pasture production. Local breeds are liable to benefit from warmer winter. In plains and dryland areas, extreme conditions like drought and water shortage may increase substantially. In areas near deserts, livestock deaths due to heat strokes may increase. In coastal zones, due to increasing temperature and sea level, the area available for grazing or fodder production may reduce. In view of climate change, adaptations to changing environment and resistance to incipient diseases will be paramount criteria in livestock production. It is liable to impact housing, feeding, health care, etc. in the livestock sector. Climate change is liable to affect disease pattern and epidemiology, ailment and fodder availability (Pilling and Hoffmann, 2011). The water scarcity for livestock production is a serious issue. The climate change is likely to aggravate water scarcity problem.

Genetic improvement and multiplication of bovine genetic resources

In India, development and improvement of indigenous breeds has been taken up by various agencies from time-to-time. These programmes had assisted in increasing the productivity of the AnGR and also helped in the conservation of indigenous germplasm. Some of the important programmes aimed at genetic improvement of livestock include National Project for Cattle & Buffalo Breeding of Deptt. of Animal Husbandry and Dairying, GOI; ICAR Network and AICRP Programmes for genetic improvement of native farm animal breeds. Presently programmes are in operation for cattle (Gir, Sahiwal, Hariana and Ongole), buffalo (Murrah, Nili Ravi, Jaffarabadi, Pandharpuri, Surti, and Bhadawari).

Genetic improvement of dairy animals depends on access to genetic variation and effective methods for exploiting this variation. With the help of the traditional breeding system, animal breeders have effectively enhanced production traits in their herds by selecting superior individuals as progenitors for the next generations, however, the genetic progress is slow, (1-3%) per year. Sustainable improvement of indigenous bovine genetic resources using New Generation Technologies and innovations coupled with traditional systems of selection is the need of the hour. Technology-driven productivity enhancement in low producing animals is the need of the hour. There is an urgent need to improve productivity, reduce inter-calving period, improve conception rates, reduce the number of services per conception.

There are many challenges in genetic improvement of dairy animals in India, mainly due to mostly small herds with non-availability of recorded data, challenging environment, low inputs, and poor management in most of the areas, uncontrolled mating, indiscriminate cross-breeding. The ambitious National Dairy Plan (NDP) was initiated in 2012 with a focus on quality dairy animal production through genetic improvement and faster multiplication of superior germplasm with strategies of improving genetic potential of bovines, producing the required number of quality bulls, and superior quality frozen semen and adopting adequate bio-security measures, etc. Further, strengthening and expanding village level infrastructure for milk procurement and provide producers with greater access to markets is also being taken care adequately under the NDP-1.

Improvement of Indigenous cattle and buffaloes could be achieved by selective breeding by incorporating modern genomic tools and production of breeding bulls, having high genetic potential, which can be achieved by utilizing progeny testing, genomic selection, and modern reproductive biotechnological tools. Modern genetic tools have to be used to increase the percentage of breedable females in milk with improved lifetime productivity. Drought resistant breeds, such as Rathi, Sahiwal, Tharparkar should be propagated in different pockets of the country having harsh climate particularly to minimize the effects of climate change. In certain areas, the productivity of dwarf breeds like Malnad Gidda, Punganur and Vechur have to be improved through selective breeding and propagated. Cross-breeding of non-descript cattle with high producing exotic cattle is recommended in the areas, where good marketing facilities for milk and milk products are available, especially in areas like Peri-urban and industrial towns, where an adequate amount of green fodder and quality feed resources exist. In India, the recommended breeds of choice for cross-breeding are Holstein and Jersey. In resource constraint areas, grading up of non-descript cattle with high genetic merit indigenous bulls, which are well-adapted to the local conditions like Sahiwal, Tharparkar, Red Sindhi, Gir, Deoni, Hariana, Ongole, Kankrej, etc. in the breeding tract is recommended (Sreenivas, 2013).

One of the major problems in buffalo improvement is out of about 54.5 million breedable buffaloes in the country; barely 15-20% are bred through AI while 80-85% is covered by natural service mostly by scrub bulls. Parentage control of breeding bulls in the buffalo improvement programmes is essential. The genetic improvement of buffalo herds in the country can be brought through selective breeding. Networking approach of progeny-testing of bulls associating multiple organized herds as well as farmer's herds, under field conditions could be followed. In certain pockets of states like Gujarat, Rajasthan, and Karnataka, Surti is recommended to be the breed of choice. Murrah is generally the breed of choice in the states of Punjab, Haryana and Western U.P., besides few pockets in Punjab, where Nili Ravi has sizable population and it also needs to be improved through selective breeding (Sreenivas, 2013). The production potential of low producing non-descript buffaloes could be increased rapidly through mating with superior sires of improved breeds like Murrah, Surti, and Mehsana. The low producing non-descript buffaloes can be replaced with relatively high producing buffaloes conforming to the characteristics of well-defined breeds through grading up with superior breeds in 5 to 6 generations (Singh and Barawal, 2010). Marker-assisted selection (MAS) and genomic selection could be utilized to select at an early age. Genetic progress can be hastened with the use of tools, such as SNP chips, high thorough-put genome sequencing, and microarray.

For many years worldwide, dairy cattle breeding programs were mainly oriented towards milk yield traits and have not given due weightage for fertility traits. In India, the main focus has been on production traits, and now the time has come to include both fertility and lifetime productivity and profitability instead of milk production alone (Ramesha and Divya, 2013). Reproductive techniques, such as multiple ovulation embryo transfers, micro-manipulation and gene transfer in the embryo; transgenesis, cloning might enable us to modify the genetic composition of an animal by means other than standard breeding techniques. The production of a calf with preferred sex is a long-cherished dream of dairy farmers. Semen can be sexed with greater than 90% accuracy with the use of a flow cytometric cell sorter. The higher cost per dose of semen combined with reduced conception rates are the limiting factors but improvements in sorting capacity, fertility, and reduction of semen cost are expected in coming years. Imported sexed semen is being used in many states.

Epilogue

Indigenous livestock have evolved over a long time in the diverse, stressful, tropical environment with adaptive traits. This situation enables them to live and endanger in these conditions. Indigenous livestock breeds are not able to compete with "improved breeds" in terms of production per se; on the other hand, they fulfill a much wider range of functions and support farming community with a wider range of quality products. The milk productivity of indigenous cattle and buffaloes could be enhanced substantially by the adoption of various modern technologies for selection and faster multiplication of genetically superior germplasm and adoption of improved animal management strategies.

References

Aggarwal, A. and Singh, M. (2006). Impact of Microclimatic modification on production of dairy animals in summer. *Indian Dairyman*, 58(3): 49-59.

Aulakh, G.S., Singla, L.D., Kaur, P. and Alka (2005). Bovine Babesiosis due to *Babesia bigemina*: Haematobiochemical and therapeutic studies. *Indian Journal of Animal Sciences.* 75(6): 617-622.

Basic Animal Husbandry Statistics. (2012, 2014, 2016). Department of Animal Husbandry, Dairying and Fisheries, Ministry of Agriculture, Government of India.

CRC Cooperative Research Centre for Beef Genetic Technologies (2006). Annual Report, 2005/2006, Armidale, NSW, Australia.

Ghosh C., Roy B., Pankaj P.K., Prasad S. and Brahma B. (2006). Management strategies to alleviate heat stress in dairy animals. *Indian Dairyman*, 58(4): 51-61.

Mwangi E.K., Stevenson P., Ndung'u J.M., Stear M.J., Reid S.W.J., Gettingby G. and Murray M. (1998). Studies on host resistance to tick infestation among Trypanotolerant *Bos indicus* cattle breeds in East Africa. *Annals of the New York Academy of Sciences* 849: 195-208.

Meuwissen, T. and M.E. Goddard, (2010). Accurate prediction of genetic values for complex traits by whole-genome re-sequencing. Genetics, 185: 623–631.

Ndungu S.G., Brown C.G. and Dolan T.T. (2005). *In vivo* comparisons of susceptibility between *bos indicus* and *bos taurus* cattle types to *Theileria parva* infection. *Journal of Veterinary Research* 72: 13-22.

Pilling, D. and Hoffmann, I. (2011). Background Study Paper No. 53. Commission on Genetic Resources for Food and Agriculture, FAO, Climate change and animal genetic resources for food and agriculture: state of knowledge, risks and opportunities.

Ramesha, K.P. (2003). Indigenous cattle and their role in this millennium, *Swadeshi Pathrike*, Page 28-32.

Ramesha, K.P. and Divya, P. (2013). Recent advances in animal genetics for enhancing dairy animal productivity in India. Paper presented in the 42nd Dairy Industry Conference, 12-14thDecember, 2013, Chennai, India.

Ramesha, K.P. and Jayaraj Rao, K. (2013). New trends in Indian Dairy Sector. CommodityIndia.com. 13(12): 23-26.

Ramesha, K.P. Jeyakumar, S., Kataktalware, M.A.. Das, D.N. Varalakshmi. S and Nagaraj, K.M. (2015). Malnad Gidda: Unique Indigenous cattle of Western Ghats, Published by the Head, SRS of ICAR-NDRI, Bengaluru-30, India, Pp: 1-116. ISBN No: 81-89650-46-7E.

Sreenivas, D. (2013). Breeding policy strategies for genetic improvement of cattle and buffaloes in India, 6(7): 455-460, doi:10.5455/vetworld.2013.455-460.

Tvedt, M.W., Hiemstra, S.J., Drucker, A.G., Louwaars, N. and Oldenborek, K. (2007). Legal aspects of exchange, use and conservation of farm animal genetic resources. FNI Report 1/2007.

Venkatachalapathy, R.T. and Iype, S. (2010). Adaptability studies on Vechur cattle of Kerala, *Proceedings of the national conference on native livestock breeds and their sustainable uses.* 27, 28 September, 2010.

❑❑❑

Chapter 2

Prospects of Genomic Selection for Improvement of Cattle and Buffaloes in India

K.P. Ramesha, P. Divya, K. Uday and R.C. Vinod

Most of the genetic progress for milk production traits in dairy animals has been made by selection on phenotype or on Estimated Breeding Values (EBV) derived from phenotype without knowledge of the number of genes that affect the trait or the effects of each gene. Over the last few years, the integration of dense genomic information into statistical tools used to make selection decisions, commonly referred to as genomic selection, has enabled gains in predicting the accuracy of breeding values for young animals without own performance. A gene map, containing at least 150 evenly spaced genetic markers along all the chromosomes, will put all genes within a detectable distance of one or two markers. Marker-assisted selection of dairy animals has become a reality and is already in use for selection of young males. Molecular genetic markers hold the key to one of the most intractable problems in animal breeding combining adaptation qualities of indigenous livestock with high productive qualities of improved exotic breeds. The power of molecular marker-assisted selection (MAS) stems from their high accuracy, increased intensity of selection and decreased generation intervals.

Genomic Selection

Genomic Selection (GS) is a form of marker-assisted selection, in which genetic markers covering the whole genome are used so that all QTL are in linkage disequilibrium with at least one marker (Goddard and Hayes, 2007). The key difference between MAS and genomic selection is that MAS concentrates on a small number of QTLs that are tagged by markers with verified associations, whereas genomic selection uses a genome-wide panel of dense markers so that all QTLs are in linkage disequilibrium with at least one marker. Genomic selection has two major advantages, first, all the genetic variance for a trait can be tracked by the marker panel. For genomic selection, one needs the reference population. This sample is analyzed to derive a prediction equation that predicts breeding value from marker genotypes, which is the genomic breeding value, such that the effect of each marker is predicted simultaneously with the other markers (Meuwissen and Goddard, 2010). Genomic selection refers to selection decisions, based on genomic breeding values (GEBV). The GEBV are calculated as the sum of the effects of dense genetic markers, or haplotypes of these markers, across the entire genome, thereby potentially capturing all the quantitative trait loci (QTL) that contribute to variation in a trait (Hayes *et al.*, 2009). The accuracy of GEBV will be achieved by both increasing the size of the reference populations and by improving the density of the SNP markers to increase the LD with QTL. Genomic selection is particularly advantageous for traits that are difficult to record at a young age. The GS procedure combines phenotype, pedigree and SNP information to arrive at Genomically Enhanced Breeding Values (GEBVs). The procedure promised to give reliabilities of GEBVs as high as 0.7 at the birth of a bull, when a large reference population of progeny tested bulls (around 20,000) is used to calculate GEBVs. The advantages of GS include a reduction in the generation interval and increased accuracy of selection at a young age, reduction in the cost of the breeding programme, tracking all the genetic variances and yields accurate effective breeding value even without phenotypic evaluation of the actual selection candidates (Dekkers, 2004; Schaeffer, 2006). GS has the potential to reduce the cost of breeding program, besides it can be used in the non-pedigreed population (Schaeffer, 2006). One of the main advantages for a country like India is genomic selection can be used in non-pedigreed populations. Genetic progress can be hastened with the use of tools, such as SNP chips, high throughput genome sequencing and microarray.

In many countries, presently, young bulls are selected based on genomic breeding values and used for AI without waiting for their progeny test results. They are also strengthening female nucleus herds and make use of ET and IVF extensively for genetic improvement. In some countries, heifers are also selected based on genomic information. Worldwide, approximately 2 million dairy cattle have now been genotyped for the purposes of genomic prediction. However, they continue to record phenotype, which is used to refine selection procedures. The possibility of selection of animals at an early stage allows defining new breeding strategies aimed at boosting genetic progress while reducing costs. In male selection in bovines, genomic selection can be used either for pre-selecting males for progeny testing (PT) or for selecting males to be used as active sires in the population. The first option produces moderate genetic gains without changing the structure of breeding programmes. The second option leads to large genetic gains, upto double those of conventional schemes because of a major reduction in the mean generation interval, but it requires greater changes in breeding programme structure. Genomic selection becomes more attractive, when it is coupled with embryo transfer technologies to further increase selection intensity on the dam-to-sire pathway.

The success of genomic selection is because of increased genetic progress on both the bull and cow genetic pathways by reducing costs compared with conventional selection schemes, but also by the potential of using this rich source of information to manage genetic resources. Genomic selection in developed countries was integrated into breeding schemes in two different ways, leading to genomic pre-selection (PS) and genomic juvenile (JS) schemes. The PS scheme entails using GEBVs to pre-select young males for PT. All subsequent steps for the selection of males remain the same as in PT schemes. Compared with PT schemes, PS schemes allow increasing the selection accuracy of young male candidates by using their genotypic information. In JS schemes, the use of genomic information is more aggressive. Although GEBVs of young sires are less accurate than conventional breeding values estimated for progeny-tested bulls, the loss in selection accuracy is compensated by a huge reduction in generation intervals, as there is no need for progeny testing. Genetic gain is then rapidly cumulated over shortened generations. In both genomic schemes, females can be genotyped to increase both accuracy and intensity for the selection of females. Genotyping both males and females is favourable in genomic dairy cattle breeding schemes (Sorensen, 2009). Phenotypic information of an indicator trait genetically, correlated with the selected trait and recorded on a large scale, can be integrated in the genomic evaluation model to improve the accuracy of predictions for traits of low heritability, when the genetic correlation between both traits is large (Calus and Veerkamp, 2011; Buch *et al.*, 2012a). GEBV reliabilities larger than 0.5 to 0.6 are already achieved in homogeneous dairy cattle populations with large reference populations (e.g. Holstein populations) for traits with moderate to high heritability (Harris and Johnson, 2010; Su *et al.*, 2010). In breeds with large effective sizes or small reference populations, the reliability of GEBVs is generally lower (0.5) even for production traits.

Commonly used Genomic Selection Methods include SNP-BLUP Method, GBLUP Method and Non-linear methods for Genomic Selection. In SNP-BLUP Method, effects of SNP is estimated in the reference population, which is genotyped and phenotyped using the statistical method. SNP effects are treated as random effects; this can be viewed as a Bayesian approach. In GBLUP Method, GEBV are estimated using phenotypes and genomic relationships, which are based on genome-wide dense marker data. A number of Non-linear methods for Genomic Selection have been developed that incorporate prior information assumes that a fraction ð of the SNPs have an effect and a fraction (1-ð) have no effect at all.

More emphasis placed on bull dam selection

In schemes integrating genomic selection, an important part of the genetic gain is achieved through the selection of bull dams (Schaeffer, 2006). Indeed, the reliability of breeding values is strongly increased for genotyped females to a level comparable with that achieved for genotyped males. Furthermore, GEBVs of bull dams are expected to be less biased, because genomic information reduces the weight attributed to own performance, which may be subject to preferential treatment. The need for large reference populations to increase GEBV accuracy has encouraged collaboration between breeding organizations and countries to exchange genotypic data (Lund *et al.*, 2011; Wiggans *et al.*, 2011). In such collaborations, all genotypes of selected and unselected candidates have to be shared to avoid biases in the estimation of genomic breeding values, at both the national and international scales (Patry *et al.*, 2011). Actually, the recent release of cheaper SNP platforms is likely to extend the use of genomic selection to a wider female population. However, before practical inclusion of female information in reference populations, the issue of preferential treatment, which frequently occurs with elite cows, must be tackled because it can introduce bias in the estimation of SNP effects, potentially decreasing the accuracy of genomic predictions.

Impact on the variability of selection response

In Progeny Testing (PT) schemes, the risk of using a bull with poor genetic merit is minimized because of PT. In PS schemes, this risk is further reduced owing to the genomic pre-selection step, which allows distinguishing with higher accuracy, the best young males within families before PT (Buch *et al.*, 2012a). In JS schemes, the accuracy of breeding values used to select AI sires is lower than that obtained after PT. Considering a fixed number of AI sires selected each year, the variability of selection response obtained by implementing a JS scheme is increased relative to conventional schemes (Buch *et al.*, 2012a). Thus, in practice, increasing the number of AI sires in JS schemes is recommended to mitigate the risk of using bulls with poor genetic merit. Another recommendation is to use young sires in 'teams' because the reliability of the mean GEBV of a group of bulls increases with group size.

New opportunities to monitor and preserve genetic diversity

Genomic selection is expected to reduce the weight of family information in selection decisions by placing the emphasis on Mendelian sampling information of young candidates (Daetwyler *et al.*, 2007). The largest reductions in inbreeding rates due to the use of genomic selection were observed for traits of low heritability (Lillehammer *et al.*, 2011) and when a large part of variance was explained by markers (de Roos *et al.*, 2011). By screening a large population of candidates, genomic selection also facilitates the identification of the least related animals, having high genetic merit with higher accuracy than before.

Defining selection objectives and integrating new selection criteria

Compared with conventional schemes, genomic selection has the potential of improving the balance of achieved genetic gain between production, conformation and functional traits. Accordingly, achieved genetic gain should better reflect economic weights considered in the total merit index (Boichard *et al.*, 2010). However, a large difference in genetic gain is still expected between highly and lowly heritable traits, if the later receive insufficient weight in the selection objective (Konig and Swalve, 2009). This phenomenon can be strengthened, if antagonistic genetic correlations exist between functional and production traits (Ytournel *et al.*, 2011). Although more complex objectives (e.g. environmental efficiency and animal welfare) are being promoted for inclusion in breeding programmes, genomic selection offers an interesting opportunity to add new selection criteria to breeding objectives (Boichard and Brochard, 2012).

Present status of genomic selection in dairy cattle breeding schemes

To date, genomic selection has only been implemented in a few countries and mainly in breeding programmes of Holstein cattle (Pryce and Daetwyler, 2012, Boichard *et al.*, 2016). The first genomic evaluations were officially released for a few Holstein populations in 2009. Different strategies have since been adopted to integrate genomic selection into existing breeding programmes. In other dairy cattle breeds, several difficulties have impeded the integration of genomic selection into breeding programmes. First, breeding programmes are generally of smaller size than Holstein programmes, which makes it more difficult to gather large reference populations. Several initiatives have, however, been created to exchange genotypes across countries, for example, the Inter-Genomics consortium for the Brown Swiss breed (Jorjani *et al.*, 2011) and the collaboration between breeding schemes of the Nordic Red Dairy cattle in Denmark, Sweden, Finland, and Norway. Second, some of these breeds may have larger effective population sizes, resulting in weaker associations between markers and QTL. Both of these factors tend to reduce the accuracy of genomic predictions, which are generally lower than in Holstein populations. The recent use of high-density SNP panels was a promising option to increase GEBV accuracy in such populations. Having large densities in SNPs reduces the physical distance between markers and QTL, and hence, should strengthen the statistical association between them. At such marker density, associations between markers and QTL may be also maintained across breeds, making it possible to build across-breed prediction equations and to capitalize on reference populations of several breeds. However, preliminary analyses of high-density chips with the genomic BLUP evaluation model only resulted in marginal gains within breeds (Su *et al.*, 2011) and across breeds (Harris *et al.*, 2011). Despite these difficulties, genomic selection has been integrated into the breeding programmes of a few large dairy cattle populations other than Holstein.

Prospects of Genomic Selection in cattle and buffaloes in India

India has some of the best breeds of cattle and buffaloes with traits for dairy, draught power, and dual purposes. Huge genetic variability exists within breeds of cattle and buffaloes of India. There is a wide gap between availability and requirement of proven dairy bulls. Among the breeding bulls in cattle, only around 20% come from organized breeding programs like progeny testing and the remaining are selected on the basis of dams yield. In the case of buffaloes, out of about 54.5 million breedable buffaloes in the country, barely 15-20 per cent is bred through AI while 80-85 per cent is covered by natural service mostly by scrub bulls. In India, the prediction equations could be made initially be based on the available records of both bulls (whose breeding values are available) and recorded females. Prediction equations developed based on a mix of a small number of progeny tested bulls and a large number of recorded females, the reliability of predicted breeding values of male calves could be raised to 35-40 per cent. Further refinement of prediction equations could be made as and when more and more records of both bulls and females are available. The impact of genomic selection is likely to be more pronounced in indigenous breeds of cattle, as the selection of males at present are solely based on mother's yield and the accuracy of selection of bulls is very low. In India, the major constraints for using GS are lack of a large number of progeny tested bulls, smallholder dairy production system and non-availability of large reference populations.

The reliability of Genomic breeding values of male calves could be raised upto 35-40 per cent, when genomic prediction equations are developed, based on reference population having a small number of progeny tested bulls (around 100) and a large number of recorded females (around 2000). Thomasen *et al.* (2014) evaluated a genomic breeding scheme in a small dairy cattle population that was intermediate in terms of using both young bulls (YB) and progeny-tested bulls (PB) and compared with a conventional progeny testing program without use of genomic information and, as the extreme case, a juvenile scheme with genomic information, where all bulls were used before progeny information was available. They reported that juvenile scheme was genetically inferior, when the increase in reliability was low (5 percentage points), but became genetically superior at higher reliabilities of genomic estimated breeding values. They further reported that juvenile scheme was always superior according to discounted profit because of the shorter generation interval and minimizing costs for housing and feeding of waiting bulls. Their report supports the use of genomic selection for cattle and buffaloes in India, as we are likely to bring about substantial genetic improvement and the genetic gains, obtained due to genomic selection will have a permanent and cumulative impact. The advantage of genomic selection includes an early and accurate selection of bull calves resulting in a higher genetic gain. In India, accuracy of selection is likely to be higher in HF / HF crossbreds than other breeds, as we can combine the information with a reference population of some of the developed countries. Genomic Selection could be highly advantageous in Indigenous breeds, where PT will not be feasible in near future. In this transition period, strategies to implement genomic selection have been rather prudent, although the largest gains could be obtained by extensive use of genomic information.

Conclusion

The success of Genomic Selection method critically depends on the availability of large databases of phenotypes and genotypes. GS also appears to be a promising tool to curb inbreeding rates because it allows exploitation of within-family genetic variance from the earliest selection stages. However, to be effective, breeders must consider using a diversified panel of genomically evaluated bulls, both to mitigate the risk of using bulls with poor merit and to limit the erosion of genetic diversity. In India, there is need and requirement of use of genomic selection for the genetic improvement of cattle and buffaloes. The actual genetic gain could be reaped by its usage for genetic improvement of indigenous cattle, where progeny testing is not possible in the near future under Indian conditions.

References

Boichard, D., Ducrocq, V., Croiseau, P. & Fritz, S. (2016). Genomic selection in domestic animals: Principles, applications and perspectives. *Comptes rendus biologies*, 339(7): 274-277.

Buch L.H., Sørensen M.K., Berg P., Pedersen L.D. and Sørensen A.C. (2012a). Genomic selection strategies in dairy cattle: strong positive interaction between use of genotypic information and intensive use of bulls on genetic gain. Journal of Animal Breeding and Genetics 129: 138–151.

Buch L.H., Kargo M., Berg P., Lassen J. and Sørensen A.C. (2012b). The value of cows in reference populations for genomic selection of new functional traits. Animal 6: 880–886.

Calus M.P.L. and Veerkamp R.F. (2011). Accuracy of multi-trait genomic selection using different methods. Genetics Selection Evolution 43: 26.

Goddard, M.E. and Hayes B.J. (2007). Genomic selection. *Journal of Animal Breeding and Genetics* 124: 323-30.

Lillehammer M., Meuwissen THE and Sonesson A.K. (2011). A comparison of dairy cattle breeding designs that use genomic selection. Journal of Dairy Science 94: 493–500.

Lund M.S., de Roos A.P.W., de Vries A.G., Druet T., Ducrocq V., Fritz S., Guillaume G., Guldbrandtsen B., Liu Z., Reents R., Schrooten C., Seefried M. and Su G. (2011). A common reference population from four European Holstein populations increases reliability of genomic predictions. Genetics Selection Evolution 43.

Schaeffer L.R. (2006). Strategy for applying genome-wide selection in dairy cattle. Journal of Animal Breeding and Genetics 123: 218–223.

Sørensen A.C. and Sørensen M.K. (2009). Genotyping both males and females is favourable in genomic dairy cattle breeding schemes. Interbull Bulletin 40: 94–97.

Thomasen J.R., Egger-Danner C., Willam A., Guldbrandtsen B., Lund M.S. and Sorensen A.C. (2014). Genomic selection strategies in a small dairy cattle population evaluated for genetic gain and profit. J. Dairy Sci. 97: 458–470.

□□□

Chapter 3

Use of Marker-based Selection Towards Genetic Improvement in Indigenous Bovines

D.N. Das and Mohan M.

Genetic improvement of a population occurs as a result of increasing the frequency of desirable genes and decreasing the frequency of the undesirable genes. Genetic progress through selection can happen regardless of the type of management, feed, or facilities used in a herd. However, the greatest genetic improvement is most likely to be realized, when animals are reared in a herd environment similar to the commercial production environment. Maintenance of good germplasm with appropriate records of either performances or pedigree always provides added advantages for selection of superior germplasm. Now-a-days, availability of genome data along with automated phenomic data of individual animal becomes easy and economical in a global scenario, which attracts future Animal husbandry for further effective manner.

How genetic improvement is achieved?

To obtain genetic improvement, the breeding value of the animals must be estimated from the measurable or quantifiable phenotypes of the animals themselves (or) those of their relatives. The phenotypes may be performance records on the prospective replacement stock, performance records on the relatives of the prospective replacement stock, or a visual evaluation of the animals or their relatives. Visual evaluation is not recommended for traits, which can be measured. In any case, there must be a mechanism in place that will permit the ranking of the tested animals from best to worst within a contemporary group for the traits under selection. A contemporary group consists of animals of the same breed and sex that were furrowed within three or four weeks of each other, housed together, fed the same feed, and managed as much alike as possible. The recommended method for comparing the genetic merit of prospective breeding animals from a contemporary group is to estimate their breeding values (EBV) or their expected progeny differences (EPD) from their own performance records and also, the performance records of their relatives. The animals with the best-estimated breeding values should be retained as replacement animals, and those with the poorest estimated breeding values should be culled from the herd. Marker Association with QTLs and genome-based selection are the latest edition in modern breeding practices in farm animals.

Genetic improvement obtained in each generation of selection depends on

The accuracy of the phenotypic evaluation(s) or the performance records decide to predict the animal's true breeding value or genotype (A). Further, accuracy indicates how well the evaluated phenotype for a particular trait relates to the animal's genotype for that trait. Accuracy is a measure of the degree of confidence that we have in the estimated or predicted breeding value. Accuracy is measured on a scale of 0 to 1, with 1 indicating an exact association between the phenotypic evaluation and the animal's true breeding value, and 0 indicates that there is no relationship between the phenotypic records and the true breeding value of the animal. Higher the accuracy, the more precisely the breeding value has been predicted. Selection accuracy helps in selecting the animals to keep as replacements for the current herd.

There is a chance of 10-30 per cent increase of accuracy of selection through gene-based and genome-based selection, if other conditions remain optimum.

The second component that determines the rate of genetic improvement is the amount of selection practised commonly called the "Selection intensity." Selection intensity for a performance trait depends on the proportion of animals that are selected relative to the total number of animals that comprise of the performance test group (contemporary group). Selection intensity (i) is the selection differential expressed in terms of phenotypic standard deviations (s); i.e. the ratio of (Ps-P) over Selection. It is used in predicting genetic response due to selection because it can be related to that per cent of the population saved as parents.

Amount of genetic or true breeding value depends on variation among animals for the trait under selection (G). Genetic variation is the variability of the genotype in the herd. An inbred herd will have a low genetic variation and therefore, will have a low rate of genetic change. Heritability is the proportion of the additive genetic variation to the total phenotypic variation. Heritability is important because without genetic variation, there will be no genetic change in the population. Alternatively, if heritability is high, genetic change can be quite rapid. Using an increasing scale from 0 to 1, a heritability of 0.75 means that 75 per cent of the total variance in a trait is controlled by additive gene action. With very high heritability, just the record of a single individual's traits can easily be used to create an effective breeding programme. Hence, genetic improvement per generation is explained as follows:

Genetic improvement/generation = A x I x G.

It is to be noted that if any one of these three factors is equal to zero, the product of the calculation is zero, indicating that no genetic progress can be expected regardless of the size of the other two factors.

The value observed while quantifying an economic trait is called the phenotypic value of that trait. Observation in terms of means, variance, the covariance of an animal population is related to phenotypic value. The partition of phenotypic value is into component attributable to the influence of genotype, environment and its interaction. The genotype is comprised of an assembly of genes possessed by the individual, and the environment depicts all non-genetic circumstances that influence the phenotypic value.

For understanding the properties of population, connected with pedigree towards the transmission of value, in terms of genetic material from parents to offspring, which cannot be done through genotypic value alone as parents pass on their genes not their genotypes to the next generation, hence a new genotype is created as a fresh in each generation. Hence, a new measure of value is required, which will refer to a gene, not the genotype. Thus, we will be enabled to assign a breeding value to the individual, a value associated with the gene carried out by the individual and transmitted to its offspring. The value associated with the gene as distinct from genotype is known as the average effect.

Natural Selection

Fitness determines the selection of a trait under natural selection. The fitness of an animal is the contribution of genes, which transmit to the next generation. Relative fitness means the fitness of an animal relative to the population mean. If the population does not expand or contract in terms of number, then the mean fitness of animals is one, where absolute fitness and relative fitness are same.

The fitness of an individual animal is the final outcome of all its developmental and physiological process. The differences between the individual in these process are seen in the variation of measurable attributes, which can be studied as metric characters. Fitness in mammals is divided into two major components *i.e.* total number of offspring and the quality of these offsprings. Hierarchy of causes of variation on metric characters under fitness reveals the viability of offspring, litter size, number of littres and milk yield and maternal behaviour.

Artificial Selection

Artificial Selection is a form of selection in which we actively choose the desirable traits, which are passed on to the offsprings. Humans have used selective breeding long before Darwin's Postulates and the discovery of genetics. Farmers chose cattle with beneficial traits, such as larger size or producing more milk, and made them breed; and although they may have known nothing about genes, they knew that the beneficial traits could be heritable.

Farmers can breed animals in order to improve productivity and thus profits. For example, dairy farmers will look for the cows that can produce more milk and those cows were only bred. These cows then pass their genes that contribute to higher milk production onto their offspring, increasing productivity in each generation for the farmers. Selection based on many traits or multi traits selection in terms of Progeny testing for male selection and Selection indices for female selection becomes effective.

Marker Assisted Selection

Genetic markers are defined as any stable and inherited variation, which is quantifiable or detectable by a suitable method and can be used subsequently to detect the presence of a specific genotype or phenotype other than itself, which otherwise is non-measurable or very difficult to detect.

In Marker-assisted selection (MAS) programme, the genetic gain is mainly increased by enhancing the accuracy of selection. However, most current animal breeding schemes are designed such that the accuracy of selection is already high *viz.* the accuracy of selection with 90 per cent in progeny testing programme. MAS is especially useful for traits, where the accuracy of conventional selection is very low, such as traits with low heritability; traits with few recording (e.g. due to expensive recoding); traits, which are measurable late in life like milk production in fifth lactation or lifetime milk production in dairy cattle and buffaloes. Further, if recordings are not available at the time of selection like slaughter quality traits or disease resistant traits that require expensive and risky challenge testing.

Hence, we reconsider the design of the conventional breeding scheme incorporating marker information, the result becomes more effective. For example, progeny testing has a high accuracy of selection with long generation interval which decreases the rate of genetic gain. MAS scheme can be designed to shorten the generation interval considerably and still maintain high accuracy of selection through the use of marker information. If we could reduce half the generation interval while maintaining the same accuracy of selection, the genetic gain could be double. Application of molecular marker for genetic improvement depends upon the ability to genotype individuals for specific genetic loci. For these purposes, three types of observable polymorphic genetic loci are generally chosen: (1) Direct markers: loci that code for the functional mutation; (2) LD markers: loci that are in population-wide linkage disequilibrium with the functional mutation; (3) LE markers: loci that are in population-wide linkage equilibrium with the functional mutation in outbred populations.

These marker loci differ not only in methods of detection but also in their application in selection programmes. While, direct markers and to a lesser degree, LD markers, allow us for selection on genotype across the population because of the consistent association between genotype with phenotype, use of LE markers generally permits different linkage phases between markers and QTL from family to family. Thus, the ease and ability to use markers in selection is opposite to their ease of detection and increases from direct markers to LD markers and LE markers. Hence, selection on these three types of markers are referred to as gene-assisted selection (GAS), LD markers assisted selection (LD-MAS), and LE marker-assisted selection (LE-MAS).

In general, current MAS scheme consists of the two steps *viz.*, statistically significant QTL(s) in a genome-wide scan for QTL consideration; and selection for these big QTL next to selecting for a new set of polygenes.

MAS nucleus scheme provides benefit, when the trait recording was before selection *e.g.* growth rate in pig or after selection *e.g.* fertility trait or milk production in dairy cattle. If the recording was before selection, MAS increased genetic gain by 8 per cent in the first generation after the start of MAS scheme. The result in terms of genetic gain was only 2 per cent after five generations. This reveals that i) extra response due to MAS is limited, when selection for traits which are also easily addressed in conventional selection scheme; ii) extra response due to MAS is reduced as the time period for selection programme becomes longer. The second one happens as both the MAS and non-MAS schemes will fix the positive QTL allele in the long-term. Hence, MAS is the difference between the two schemes will further become small in the long-term period. MAS opens a way to increase short-term gains. This will still yield continuous benefits in ongoing MAS schemes, as new QTL are being detected continuously.

Genomic Selection

For QTL identification, we perform both molecular and statistical association analysis to explain a limited fraction of the genetic variation in the population. Further, all QTLs cannot be taken into consideration, if there is a lack of linkage association. Hence, an alternative procedure in which the entire genome of an individual is considered and all genes across the chromosomes explain the variation and functional effects on the traits designed to be selected. To avoid non-additive genetic effects, the knowledge of conventional breeding tools can also be incorporated with necessary modification to reduce generation interval.

Genetic gain due to Genomic Selection

After seven years of genomic selection in the United States by USDA, the impact of this technology on the population was estimated. Selection differential(s) (SD) and generation interval(s) (GI) were calculated based on four-path selection model, which includes sire(s) of bulls (SB), sire(s) of cows (SC), dam(s) of bulls (DB), and dam(s) of cows (DC) pathways. Changes in SD over the period of time were estimated for milk, fat, and protein yield; somatic cell score (SCS);

productive life (PL); and daughter pregnancy rate (DPR) traits for the Holstein Friesian breed. After the implementation of genomic selection, significant reductions were observed in GI, especially the SB and SC pathways. GI in the SB path reduced from 7 years to less than 2.5 years, and the GI of the DB path declined from about 4 years to nearly 2.5 years. Whereas, GI of SD path was relatively stable for yield traits. Further, through this path, modest genetic gains were observed. Response to selection was significantly influenced due to genomic approach for lowly heritable traits like DPR (daughters pregnancy rate), PL(productive lifespan), and SCS (somatic cell score). There was a significant change in genetic trend from close to zero to large and favourable, resulting in a rapid genetic improvement in fertility, lifespan, and health traits. This clearly indicated that genomic selection contributed significantly towards genetic improvement in dairy cattle in the USA. Application of genomic selection through four-path selection model revealed that the genetic gain per year increased from 50 to 100 per cent for milk yield traits and from 3 to 4 - fold for lowly heritable traits.

Production traits like milk yield, fat and protein yields traits revealed varying economic trends in the net merit. The genetic improvement was expected, as these traits are with moderate heritability. Similar genetic trend was observed over a period of time in milk yield and protein yield, as they were highly correlated (r=0.93). Due to high selection pressure through sire paths (SB & SC), in which very best bulls are used for high selection differential (SD). Genomic selection has produced a significant increase in milk yield in short-term in all paths except DC. The cows revealed a genetic gain of milk, protein and fat yield as 58, 2.6 and 1.8 kg per year prior to genomic selection, which increased twice due to a post-genomic selection effect (109, 6.0 and 4.1).

Though the lower h^2 for PL was recorded as 0.08 and selection accuracy was found to be low for young animals, which have few offsprings with direct culling information, after application of genomic selection, it was observed that this lowly heritable trait contributed around 22 per cent towards an economic index of net merit. A substantial increase in SD in sire of bulls (SB), sire of cows (SC), and dam of bulls (DB) pathways. The annual genetic gain was reported to be 4 to 15 - folds for all paths (SB, SC, DB, DC).

Genetic evaluation of SCS in the USA is carried out since 1994. This trait has the most reliable relationship between the presence of clinical and subclinical mastitis. From 1985 to 2000, no clear trends in any of the four paths (SB, SC, DB, SC) was noticed. Selection differential of SCS from 2000 to 2015 was higher in population in relation to SB, SC, and DB. Annual genetic gain through four paths of selection was about 330 per cent increase in SCS.

Daughter pregnancy rate (DPR) is the measure of the ability of daughter of a bull to become pregnant and presently receive 11 per cent of the emphasis in lifetime total merit. The gradient of positive direction represents the higher-level fertility in cows. Being lowly heritable trait, there is a limited scope of improvement through conventional breeding. It remains as a negative gradient throughout 30 years of selection, as there is genetic antagonism in milk yield and fertility. There was a steady increase in selection differential of this trait through SC and DB paths.

Future strategies required for cattle and buffalo improvement under field conditions

For genetic improvement towards sustainable improvement of cattle and buffaloes with the aim of financial and socio-economic development of farmers, salient strategies are necessary to adapt to face the major challenges under climate change scenario are as follows:

Application of unified co-coordinating (Govt. Co-operative and corporate with Govt. support) mechanism for breeding programmes with the maintenance of conventional inventories and online database, which can be maintained at village Panchayat; Block/Taluka, followed by District and State level with close contact with Central Government for centralized storage of data on Animal genetic resources. Performance recordings including milk quality; udder health; general health of animals for each breed of cattle and buffaloes for selection of elite male and females; replacement of stock and dissemination of proven germplasm under field conditions. Long-term breeding policies and strategies with a projection of requirement of breeding inputs. Protection of true breed; elite germplasms under field conditions can be encouraged by Dairy Mela; awarding farmers; formation of Breeders' Association and by the implementation of rules to avoid indiscriminate breeding. Genetic improvement programmes in draught breeds should also be targeted, as they are available in good in numbers in different geographical location.

Table 1: Molecular marker tests used in commercial breeding for different species

Trait category	Direct marker	Linkage Equilibrium marker	Linkage Disequilibrium marker
Congenital defects	BLAD (D) Citrulinaemia (D,B) DUMPS (D) CVM (D) Maple syrup urine (D,B) Mannosidosis (D,B) RYR (P)	RYR (P)	Polled (B)
Appearance	CKIT (P) MC1R/MSHR (P,B,D) MGF (B)		
Milk Quality	κ-Casein (D) β-Lactoglobulin (D) FMO3 (D)		
Meat Quality	RYR (P) RN/PRKAG3 (P) >15 PICmarq (P)	RYR (P) RN/PRKAG3 (P) A-FABP/FABP4 (P) H-FABP/FABP3 (P) CAST(P, B) THYR (B) Leptin (B)	
Feed intake	MCAR (P)		
DISEASE	Prp (S) F18 (P)	B blood group (C) K88 (P)	
Reproduction	Booroola (S) Inverdale (S) HannaB (S)	Booroola (S) ESR (P) PRLR (P) RBP4 (P)	
Growth and composition	MC4R (P) IGF-2 (P) Myostatin (B) Callipyge (S)	CAST (P) IGF-2 (P) Carwell (S)	QTL (P) QTL (B)
Milk yield and composition	DGAT (D) GRH (D) κ-Casein (D)	PRL (D)	QTL (D)

D: dairy cattle; B: beef cattle; C: poultry; P: pigs; S: sheep (Dekkers, 2004)

- Easily recordable traits like daily milk yield, lactation milk yield, body condition score, functional survival trait (cows' ability to remain in the herd for the functional reasons like sound health irrespective productive and reproductive performances).
- The mechanism for monitoring of focal points (AI centres, sperm stations, farms, breeding programme, etc.). Monitoring cell for certification of sperm stations and AI bulls including sourcing and use of quality bulls for breeding is necessary to apply very effectively.

- Optimum and effective utilization of fodder and feed resources both in qualitative and quantitative terms.
- Adoption of a dynamic HRD strategy reflecting manpower requirements at central/State levels and the need for skill up-gradation.
- Legislative backup for standardization and certification of semen stations or for identification and recording of the animals in the milk pockets.
- Threshold Somatic cell count and genetic/major disease investigation could be immediate targets for sustainability of milk production, especially in indigenous cattle and buffaloes.
- Insurance coverage, both for livestock and farmers, are necessary to address.

References

Beuzen *et al.* (2000). Molecular markers and their use in animal breeding. The veterinary Journal. 160: 42-52.

Dekkers, J.C.M. (2004). Commercial application of marker- and gene-assisted selection in livestock: Strategies and lessons. *J. Anim. Sci.* 82: E313-28

Falconer, D.S. and Mackay, T.F.C. (2013). Introduction to Quantitative Genetics (4th edition).

Meuwissen, T., Hayes, B., and Goddard, M. (2013). Accelerating improvement of livestock with genomic selection. Annu. Rev. Anim. Bioscie. 2013. Jan; 1: 221-37.

Weller, J.I. (2007). Current and future developments in patents for quantative trait loci in dairy cattle. Recent patents on DNA & gene sequences. 1: 69-76.

❏❏❏

Chapter 4

Role of Genomics for Selection of Disease Tolerant Bovines

D.N. Das

Infectious disease is a major challenge to bovine breeders. Economic losses due to infectious diseases in livestock production system are accounted around 20 per cent in developed countries and 35-50 per cent in developing countries, respectively. However, the true cost of disease incidence and management is a complex phenomenon. Zoonotic diseases like Tuberculosis, Rabies, Brucellosis, Anthrax, *etc.* are important from both human and animal health point of view. The incidence of infectious diseases like mastitis and FMD impedes the growth of the dairy industry, despite widespread application of antibiotics, vaccines, quarrantine, & other conventional disease control measures. Technological inventions in the area of animal health open up new avenues for detection, management, control and eradication of diseases. The impact of these innovations extends beyond the boundary of animal health and welfare, and could significantly contribute to improving human health and food security.

There is the presence of thousands of known associations between genetic variants and complex phenotypes of human or animal, and the rate of novel discoveries is rapidly increasing. Transformation of these associations into the knowledge of disease mechanisms remains a fundamental challenge because the associated variants are mostly in non-coding regions of the genome, where there are limited guiding principles to predict their functions. Based on identified genetic associations with maps of regulatory activity across the human genome has revealed that phenotype-associated variants are highly enriched in candidate regulatory elements. Hence, allele-specific analysis of gene regulation can further select variants, which likely have a functional effect on disease mechanisms. Newly discovered high-throughput assays to quantify the activity of candidate regulatory elements are way forward for disease diagnosis and control.

Noble control of infection in livestock is genetic disease resistance, the inherent capacity of a previously unexposed animal to resist a virulent challenge. Genomics has opened a new avenue in disease investigation and vaccine research in livestock. So far, genetic selection of animals placed emphasis on productivity and efficiency, which has potentially reduced natural disease resistance. It is now appropriate to implement these combined efforts of genomics with conventional breeding practices for selection of superior dairy animals to bring cost-effective and faster genetic improvement. Classical genetic selection, recently aided by genomic selection tools becomes successful in achieving remarkable progress in dairy animal improvement.

Selection of superior dairy animals, based on true genetic merit or breeding value is the main key to their genetic improvement. Genetic improvement is decided based on two principal components *viz.* (a) the existence of variability in the population (b) the population, which is heritable, i.e. the heritability. Success for selection also depends on having clear, well-defined objectives, which support selection through replacing less desirable alleles by better alleles in the population. The genetic progress is the product of the intensity of selection times, the heritability of the trait under selection times, the phenotypic standard deviation of that trait. If any of these three parts is low, genetic progress through selection will be slow. The economic value of the trait may still justify efforts to improve it through selection; as such improvement is a permanent change that benefits all future offspring. Heritability helps the dairy producer to decide which traits justify improvement through selection. Heritability is one important component of the equation used to predict genetic progress from selection to improve a trait.

Resistance to disease development is classified into three categories: (1) Complete level of tolerance: This indicates no-development of disease, (2) True tolerance: It is defined as the ability of an animal to maintain a reasonable level of productivity, when it is diseased, (3) Resilience: Which is ability of the affected individuals to require minimal treatment to maintain acceptable performance. In a study, in Holstein Friesian cows, Schukken *et al.* (1999) reported that 20.7 per cent of Holstein cows experimentally challenged with the same dose of *S. aureus* Newbould 305 that did not establish infection in any of the quarters, whereas, 20 per cent had all quarters infected.

Selection based on immune responsiveness for better health

The High Immune Response (HIR) evolved by the University of Guelph determines the cows or calves with the best immune responses. It is established that cows with optimal immune responses or HIR cows exhibited less occurrence of disease, improved milk, and colostrum quality, and respond better to vaccination. In fact, HIR cows were found to be with 30 to 60 per cent reduction in economically important diseases like mastitis, metritis, displaced abomasums, retained fetal membrane and are less likely to be seropositive for Johne's disease. Further, these associations represent substantial benefits for herd health management and better longevity, which results in direct-cost savings. Hence, it is better to identify HIR cows in the herd for future genetic improvement programme.

Immune response traits are heritable, approximately with 0.25 heritability, indicating that 25 per cent of the variation in these traits is attributed to the cow's genetics. This heritability is similar to milk production traits indicating that similar genetic gain for immune response traits would be possible, as it is obtained for these production parameters. Breeding for overall immune response is likely to provide protection against a multitude of diseases since antibody-mediated immune response (AMIR) and cell-mediated immune response (CMIR) provide tolerance against diverse micro-organisms of either extra-cellular or intra-cellular pathogens in nature. As heritability of resistance for a particular disease is quite low (<0.10), so, breeding for immune response overcomes problems associated with breeding for resistance to a particular disease. Finally, it is possible to bring significant and rapid genetic gain by breeding for enhanced immune response.

Role of Genomics for Host-Pathogen Interaction

Dairy farmers face challenges every day whether to decide to keep and treat or cull an animal. Dairy producers choose to market dairy cattle for a number of reasons, whether reproduction, poor milk quality, low milk production, lameness or a number of other possibilities. Studies show that 26.7 per cent of producers culled cattle because of reproductive issues, making it the most prevalent reason for culling dairy cattle. Producers with a good reproductive programme create an optimal dairy environment, managing income losses caused by long days open and reducing reproductive culling.

Economic analysis shows that calving intervals extended beyond 13 months result in reduced annual revenue. Studies revealed that high somatic cell counts (SCC) have a dramatic effect on reproductive efficiency. Even, cows with chronic metabolic disorders after calving can cause long-term damage to the reproductive tract, resulting in infertility. Damage to the uterus may lead to difficult calving. Further, the higher the number of services per conception, the less fertile the animal is. Each day cows stay open past the voluntary waiting period costs the dairy producer money.

An economic analysis conducted recently indicated that regardless of the use of rBST, an extended calving interval of more than 13 months results leading to loss of annual revenue per cow. It is more profitable, if more often a cow becomes pregnant during its productive lifetime. If producers are having a difficult time getting cows re-bred and cows are freshening with greater than a 16-months calving interval, culling is advantageous compared to the additional costs of housing, care, and feed, when cattle are not bred and are producing a lesser quantity of milk.

One of the major objectives of the host response to infectious diseases is to discover novel components of the host immune system critical to robust host defense. Identification of these components at the molecular level is the first step to understand how the host reacts with the infectious challenge and builds a foundation, which determines rational therapies or vaccine design for augmentation of host resistance.

The interaction between host and pathogen leading to infection is multi-dimensional, dynamic and exceedingly complex. Hence, there is a necessity for a thorough understanding of pathogenesis of a given infection, which includes a complete inventory of the spatial and temporal expression of genes by both the host and pathogen from the time of exposure to the final resolution of infection considering the potentially large number of factors that influence the host defense, precise identification of gene is a formidable challenge.

For studying the host-pathogen interactions and the role of genomics for disease occurrence, commercially available inbred strains of mice are used under animal model through well-defined infection challenge. Correlation of the inheritance of susceptibility or resistance to a specific infectious challenge with one or more chromosomal regions is then performed by linkage analysis. Finally, known genes within the genetic architecture must be evaluated and novel genes must be positionally cloned to elucidate the underlying molecular basis of the immune defense. Comparative genomic analysis is a logical extension of these principles. Knowledge of the genomic organization of the bovine orthologues of susceptibility genes identified through the experimental challenge. These genes can then be tested as candidates for disease susceptibility through mutation analysis.

Candidate genes governing resistance against Production diseases

Mastitis is an inflammation of the mammary gland, caused by infection, by more than 150 types of micro-organisms. Pathogens causing mastitis are classified into major and minor pathogens. Major pathogens are mostly responsible for infection and include contagious pathogens, such as *Staphylococcus aureus* and *Streptococcus agalactiae,* which reside pre-dominantly in the udder and spread during milking, and pathogens, which are present in the environment are mainly coliforms, and *enterococci.*

Host defense mechanisms against udder infection involve morphological and physiological characteristics and responses of the immune system. Immune system defense mechanism includes innate and adaptive mechanisms. Although innate and adaptive mechanisms are intimately linked, innate immunity is non-specific and generally includes an influx of polymorphonuclear neutrophils (PMN) and macrophages, which are released from the blood into mammary tissue upon infection, and production of soluble components, such as peroxides, lysozyme, lactoferrin, and complement components.

Adaptive immunity is specific to a pathogen and it involves antibody formation by B-cells, helper T-cell, and cytotoxic functions. T-cells are activated through the T-cell receptor complex, following recognition of antigen in association with MHC molecules. Activation of T-helper and T cytotoxic cells is modulated by recognition of BoLA-class II and class I molecules, respectively. It is critical to realize that the importance of the various host defense mechanisms can differ by pathogen and may change during infection. For instance, aspects of innate host resistance may predominate during *E. coli* mastitis, which tends to be short-term, whereas B- and T cell activity may be more relevant in later stages of infection. Bacterial infection and the resulting host responses result in a variety of compositional changes in milk. Several of these immunological parameters are used as indicators or markers of mastitis, most importantly somatic cell count (SCC), which measures the concentration of leucocytes (mainly PMN) in milk.

Besides managemental control for disease either against specific infection like mastitis, metritis, viral infection like FMD, or parasitic, fungal infestation, it is necessary to understand that host genome interaction, which is controlled by a number of candidate genes like NRAMP1, MHCII DRB3, DQA, DQB, Interleukin, TLR2, TLR4, HSP1AI, BTN1A1, Lactoferrin, PRL, *etc.* through various functional pathways. Hence, selection of farm animals based on desirable allelic combination with respect to disease resistance in association with growth, production and reproduction performances is very much important towards the creation of disease-tolerant livestock. Further, new approaches in Whole Genome Sequencing and deep Proteomics profiling of livestock for genetic improvement of economically important traits are new areas for creation disease tolerant livestock. Genetic engineering plays a parallel role for studying and improving diseases tolerant phenomenon and production of disease-tolerant farm animals.

Genomic selection in Dairy animals

Genomic selection is now replacing the conventional methodology of genetic evaluation in dairy cattle. Genomic selection thought to be superior to marker-assisted selection. Unlike marker-assisted selection, based on data on only tens of genetic markers, genomic selection is based on associating thousands of genetic-markers spread over the genomes of several thousand animals.

The end result is the estimate of the association between each marker and each phenotype. With the invention of genotyping platforms with individual detection elements capable of simultaneously assaying upto 777,000 distinct SNP genetic-markers, which are evenly distributed across the bovine genome are now commercially available (Illumina Inc., San Diego, CA). Whole genome sequencing on a large number of animals once becomes feasible, a number of useful markers will be used dramatically.

Once each marker effect is known, then an animal without its functional phenotype e.g., a disease-free newborn calf can be genotyped and its direct genomic value (DGV) can be estimated, based on the genotype only. This is generally integrated with the traditional genetic evaluation method to generate a genomic-estimated breeding value (GEBV). The advantage of such a method to achieve accurate estimates of genetic merit through exploiting knowledge of the genotype of the animal, even if the animal is very young.

Production of Disease resistant genetically modified (GM) Animal

Disease control strategies mainly depend on both the pathogen and the host. Conventionally, control of animal disease involves either destruction of the pathogen or the vector carrying the pathogen, through vaccination, treatment using antibiotics and other drugs, or spraying disinfectants to kill mosquitoes. Despite the success of these conventional strategies in combating specific diseases, there are many continuing challenges relating to animal health and disease. Further, due to indiscriminate use of antibiotics, anthelmintic, *etc.*, pathogens get resistant and genome gets mutated and evolve in such a way that the control strategy no longer becomes effective. In India, recently, control of dengue, malaria, and chikunguniya become cumbersome due to mutation of genome structure of causative agents.

As an alternative to conventional approaches, powerful genetic tools are becoming available to assist in combating the disease. Wild species of herbivores were domesticated by humans, few thousands of years back. These species were genetically modified for our own purposes indirectly through selection. To a large extent, the huge differences between today's livestock and their ancestors are a testament to how successful selection and genetic improvement happened. Animals were selected on observable phenotypes without understanding the molecular mechanism of inheritance. With the advent of molecular tools along with advanced Animal breeding and computational tools desirable genotypes, controlling the economic traits of farm animals can be selected for future genetic improvement.

Although traits, such as fertility and disease resistance are still difficult to quantify and improve. In the conventional breeding process, for selection of desirable characters like growth, production, etc. Some undesirable traits viz. poor reproductive performance and lower resistance against disease are automatically incorporated. In addition, QTLs present in the parents is transmitted in the next generation for selection of superior progenies, which severely limits the range and extent of genetic improvement. To overcome these limitations, gene addition through transgenic technology potentially opens a new vista. Genetic modification offers alternative strategies for conventional animal breeding. This technology can be applied for a specific application, where genetic variation does not exist significantly in a population towards holistic genetic improvements programme. With this approach, there is a possibility to enhance the ability of the animals to mount an appropriate immune response against the pathogen or to generate an effective system, which would directly block the entry of pathogen and destroy them. Further, a combination of strategies may prove to be the most successful approach.

The *Mx* genes of vertebrates were first discovered in mice due to the presence of functional alleles for induction of a potent anti-viral state in response to infection by specific groups of viruses including influenza probably due to interferon-induced anti-viral mechanisms.

Herman bull, world's first genetically modified transgenic bovine in 1990. Researchers carried out transgenic work through micro-injection in cells at an early embryonic stage with a human gene coding for lactoferrin. Eight calves were born in 1994 and all offsprings modified lactoferrin gene. Further, 83 offsprings were born to this elite bull. In 2011, GM dairy cows were produced by Chinese and Argentina scientists. Objectives of these studies were to produce genetically modified cow milk, which resembles like human breast milk, as genes from human milk were introduced. In 2012, scientists from New Zealand also developed a genetically engineered cow that produced allergy-free milk. Similarly, genetically modified polled Holstein Friesian dairy cow was developed through gene editing at Red Angus breed of cattle. A short strip of DNA was taken from the genome of Red Angus breed, in which genes suppress horn growth.

Potential of GM technology towards genetic improvement of novel economic traits of livestock can be generated. There are two advantages of using genetically modified (GM) livestock in our society. First, the GM animals could be used for a model for studies on disease progression and its control. In this situation, it is likely that relevant information related to human disease may also be gathered indirectly. Secondly, GM based disease-resistant livestock and their produce could be used in the food chain.

a) Dominant-negative proteins

Dominant negative mutants have already provided information into the molecular mechanisms of action of a number of protein families like hormone receptors, oncogenes, and growth factor receptors, and it was also identified for the cause few autosomal dominant diseases. Further, expression of dominant negative mutants under the control of highly active lung cell-specific promoters provides strong support to the study of the roles of specific-proteins and protein families in lung development, health, and disease. Introduction of mutant key factors in pathogen infection like cell surface receptors can block disease progression. Interaction of parasite with surface molecules on mammalian host cells initiates host cell responses, which significantly controls the progress of the infection. The Abl family of protein kinases and also, PKR are non-receptor protein kinases and play a pivotal role in determining the outcome of *Leishmania* infestations.

b) Ribonucleic acid interference (RNAi)

This method enables the ability of specific short RNA sequences to anneal with the RNA of the pathogen, causing the destruction of the foreign RNA. RNAi requires access to the target RNA, which may limit this approach to viruses. Mechanism of silencing gene expression through RNA interference (RNAi) towards activating the RNAi pathway is useful for its application to enhance livestock production through increased production efficiency and prevention of disease.

RNAi technology is applied to study the role of oncogene expression in leukaemia cell lines and to validate the therapeutic potential of RNAi for treatment of blood disorders. Due to rapid globalization, and changing climate scenario, there is an ascending trend of transmission of infectious diseases, including avian influenza, severe acute respiratory syndrome (SARS), and swine influenza, *etc.* Hence, the prevention of these diseases is necessary. Gene silencing technologies including antisense oligonucleotide (ASO), RNA interference (RNAi) and single strand-small interfering RNA (ss-siRNA) could be a better and effective choice for controlling diseases. The primary mechanism of this noble technology is to inhibit gene expression and destroy specific RNA molecule of the pathogen. Use of gene silencing tool is expected to give a new alternative for effective eradication of infectious diseases in animals and humans.

c) Ribonucleic acid decoys

Short strands single-stranded RNA can mimic mRNA sequences and compete for proteins, which act as translational activators and stabilize mRNA. These RNA decoys are potentially attractive and useful. Expression of RNA sequences, which mimic specific sequences within a pathogen can disrupt the activity of the pathogen's replication machinery. Again, this approach is probably restricted to specific viruses like influenza causing virus.

Recently, the role of both short and long non-coding RNAs (ncRNAs) for regulation of gene expression has drawn significant attention. Non-coding RNA-based regulation is achieved through a variety of mechanisms, in which some are relatively well-understood, while others are not much clear. MicroRNAs (miRNAs) being endogenous small RNAs regulate gene expression in eukaryotic organisms. Currently, it is noticed that role for long ncRNAs i.e. miRNA decoys, also referred to as target mimics or sponges, in which long ncRNAs carry a short stretch of sequence sharing homology to miRNA-binding sites in endogenous targets. As a result, miRNA decoys enable to sequester and inactivate miRNA function. Engineered miRNA decoys are also efficient and useful tools for studying gene function. For disease detection and control, this technology is a new precise approach.

Conclusion

Selection of suitable disease tolerant breeds of dairy animals suited to present climate change environment for sustainable production and reproduction performances towards maximizing profitability based on conventional, molecular, reproductive and GM based technologies could be the choice for future genetic improvement programme. Biopharma, along with personalized medicines, may bring the new concept for health management of animals and humans, in which knowledge of omics will be useful to make 'One health concept' successful.

References

Berry D.P, Kearney J.F. and Harris B.L. (2009). Genomic selection in Ireland. Interbull Bulletin. Uppsala Sweden, 29-34.

C.B.A. Whitelaw and H.M. Sang, (2005). Disease-resistant genetically modified animals. *Rev. Sci. Tech. Off. Int. Epiz.*, 24(1): 275-283.

Stephen C. Bishop and John A. Woolliams, (2014). Genomics and disease resistance studies in livestock *Livestock Science* 166: 190–198.

D.N. Das and Sapna Nath, (2015). Somatic Cell Count (SCC): An indicator for detection of quality milk and milk products. Paper presented at the National Seminar on Quality- A Tool for value addition of dairy foods, Bangalore, 23-24 January, 2016.

D.N. Das, (2014). 'Functional genomics in productive and reproductive health' Paper presented in Winter School "Advanced concepts and techniques to augment reproduction in livestock" NIANP, Bengaluru, 12th Nov., 2014 - 2nd Dec., 2014.

Dekkers, J.C.M., and F. Hospital, (2002). The use of molecular genetics in the improvement of agricultural populations. *Nat. Rev. Genet.* 3: 22–32.

❑❑❑

Chapter 5

Conservation of Animal Genetic Resources: Problems and Prospects

D.N. Das and Mohan M.

Charles Darwin is one of the most important personalities of the science of the last five hundred years. In his book, on the Origin of Species by Means of Natural Selection, or the Preservation of Favoured Races in the Struggle for Life, published in 1859, Darwin proposed what is now called the Theory of Evolution. This book, along with its best-known companion The Descent of Man, and Selection in Relation to Sex, published in 1871, precipitated a major change in scientific thinking about the origin of life, particularly in the field of biology.

Epigenetics and Evolution

Epigenetics interestingly occupies a pivotal role in the concept of inheritance, natural selection and, perhaps, even evolution. The great science philosopher Karl Popper opined that "we should altogether avoid, like the plague, discussing the meaning of words." Literature revealed that epigenetics is to explain changes in gene expression. Other schools of thoughts use it to refer to trans-generational effects and/or inherited expression states. This disagreement on a clear definition has made it difficult for the synthesis of epigenetic research across fields.

Intra-generational epigenetics deals with the modification of gene expression through epigenetic markers like DNA methylation, covalent histone modification, micro RNA action, *etc.* which results into a modified phenotype, often at the molecular/cellular level, within an individual's lifespan. That's why, we use the terminology as "the epigenetics of cancer" or "epigenetics of cardiovascular disease", *etc.*

Transgenerational epigenetics describes the inheritance of a modified phenotype from the parental generation without changes in genes or gene sequence. Epigenetic markers, as mentioned above may be responsible, but a focus in this category is on the act of inheritance. Some authors used the restrictive term "cross-generational" to identify inherited traits resulting from the direct exposure of gametes of the F_1 and F_2 generations while within the body of the P_0 generation.

Breed

A breed is a subspecific group of domestic livestock with definable and identifiable external characteristics that enable it to be separated by visual appraisal from other similarly defined groups within the same species or a group for which geographical and/or cultural separation from phenotypically similar groups has led acceptance of its separate identity (FAO, 2012). The breed is adapted in a specific geographical location over a period of time through natural or artificial selection. Further, the breed is to be registered under-recognized registration organization in a country and published worldwide.

Future of Breed

Criteria for endangerment of a breed

A breed is declared to be endangered, if the available number of animals for future breeding is minimized below a certain level. Further, individual animals maintained at different localities will not provide a guarantee for the continuation of a breed, if they are not allowed to take part in the process of reproduction and also, by the ratio of dams and sires. A determining factor termed as effective population size, Ne is calculated as per the following formula:

$$N_e = [4 \times N_m \times N_f]/[N_m + N_f]$$

Where, N_m represents the number of available male animals

and N_f represents the number of available female animals

The effective population size, N_e can also be utilized for calculation of inbreeding, DF per generation with the following formula:

$$DF = \Delta N_e$$

For a successful selection of economic traits like body size, body weight, etc., an effective population size of more than 100 animals is required. The effective population size of 50 may also be considered for selection and breeding programme. The consequent rise in inbreeding depression at the rate of 1 per cent is acceptable. The data, presented in Table 1, reveals an equal strength of dams and sires if used in the breeding programme. Although practically not always feasible, the inbreeding depression will be 0.5% after one generation. Under normal circumstances, the number of series will always be lower than the number of dams but even than 20 sires and 50 dams will be sufficient (Brem *et al.*, 1989).

Table 1: Determination of effective population size and inbreeding co-efficient based on sire to dam ratio

Males (n)	Females (n)	Total (n)	Effective population size (Ne)	Increase in inbreeding after one generation (%)
50	50	100	100	0.5
20	80	100	64	0.78
10	90	100	36	1.39
1	99	100	3.96	12.63
20	50	70	57.1	0.88
10	50	60	33.3	1.50
1	50	51	3.92	12.75

Risk status of the indigenous breed

In India, out of 37 indigenous cattle and 13 buffalo breeds reported in Breed Wise Survey conducted during 2013, eight cattle breeds (nearly 21.42%) and 2 buffalo breeds were at risk status. Breeds like Mewati, Ponwar, Siri, Bargur belong to vulnerable status, as the population is within 10,000 to 20,000. Vechur, Punganur, Pulikulam, Krishna Valley breeds of cattle Chilika & Toda breeds of buffaloes were at endangered status, as their population is within 1000 to 10,000 in nos.

Present scenario in India

Presently, there are 41 recognized cattle and 13 buffalo breeds in India. Among milch breeds, Gir, Sahiwal, Red Sindhi are important. Deoni, Ongole, Hariana, Tharparker, and Kankrej are prominent dual-purpose cattle breeds of our country. Among draught breeds, Hallikar, Amritmahal, Khillari, Kangayam, Gaolao, etc. are the major breeds of cattle. There are certain breeds of cattle, which are dwarf in nature and play a significant role in the agricultural economy of the regions and have special characteristics. The numbers of Vechur, Krishna Valley and Punganur breeds are significantly low at their native tracts. During 19th century (1849-1854), native cattle of India is popularly known as Brahman cattle probably comprising of Gir, Ongole, Nellore and Krishna Valley were imported to USA, Mexico, Brazil, breeds were improved through selective breeding as well as cross-breeding with the intention of better beef production.

As per Livestock Census, 2007 and 2013 Haryana cattle forms a major portion of the registered cattle population, followed by Gir. About 40 per cent of the registered draft breeds population declined. Murrah buffalo and its grades contribute nearly 50 per cent of the total buffalo population and there is a rapid increase in its population from around 20 million to 50 million in 2013 than the previous census (2007). This clearly indicates that the farmers' interest shifted towards nurturing more milch and dual-purpose indigenous breeds to meet the requirement of milk production than dwarf breeds as mechanization of agriculture system prevails in rural India and delay in earning due to value added services like organic farming through draft and dwarf breeds of cattle.

The Utility of Conservation

The need for preservation and propagation of domesticated animals for their genetic improvement with eco-friendly maintenance of biodiversity is well-known to modern society. It has been discussed since the First World Congress on Applied Genetics in Madrid, in 1974. The breeds are classified as insecure, vulnerable, endangered or critical. The Food and Agriculture Organization (FAO) has provided the guidelines for assessing the survival risk, if the population size approaches the number of five thousand. Due to the extensive breed substitution and continuous cross-breeding practices in the past many "unproductive" animal species have been neglected and are facing extinction at an alarming rate. In November 1993, FAO published the first "World Watch List for Domestic Animal Diversity" and warned that many breeds of domestic animals are becoming extinct at an accelerating rate of 50 per year or around one per week.

The former FAO Director-General once stated that "The rich diversity of cultivated livestock breeds patiently developed by generations and adapted to their need for millennia is vanishing at an alarming pace. For the sake of higher returns, the stockbreeding of intensive production has been developed, which focuses naturally only on certain highly productive breeds. We have to protect, conserve and output for better use of the vast reservoir of diversity, offered by nature and traditional forms of agriculture".

Conservation methods followed in India are as follows

***In-situ* conservation:** Conservation of the breed is practiced at its own breeding tracts:

1. Implementation of National Breeding Policy: Based on National Breeding policy in the direction of the recommendation of National Agricultural Commission, following strategies were considered:
   - Development of the Nationwide awareness about breed conservation with special emphasis on not to cross the registered breed with exotic or crossbred.
   - For the creation of scope for indigenous breed usage, the state government should implement the policy so that the non-descript population can be graded up with the regional specific breeds to promote the farmers to rear indigenous animals.
   - Supply of superior germplasm of the indigenous breeds at farmer doorstep through network projects.
2. Promotion of Breeders' Organisation: This will help animal conservation and also, establish a legal framework to govern cattle handling as well as the purchase of animals in India and also, a large data generation centre through National Grid so that conservation and improvement of a specific breed will be easy at field level.
3. Enhancing of Volunteer NGOs' to Promote the Concept of Goshalas/Goushadans/Pinjarpore: Organizations, which promote conser-vation of bovine and buffalo genetic resources should be encouraged to preserve the germplasm with sufficient care in terms of breeding, feeding and management with the co-operation of Agricultural Universities, ICAR Institutes and local Veterinary and Animal Husbandry Departments.

Ex-situ Conservation

The conservation of biological diversity outside its natural habitat including live animal conservation (*In-vivo*) and cryopreservation of germplasm in gene banks (In-vitro).

***In-vivo*:** Conservation of animals is executed at organized government farms, breeding farms, semen stations, etc.

***In-vitro*:** Cryopreservation of the sperm, ova, embryo, reproductive organs, DNA, *etc.* are carried out at regional as well as at the national level.

Assistant Reproduction Techniques (ART)

These modern techniques help to recreate or improve breed number over a period of time. Most common techniques, which are practice successfully in India are as follows:

- **Artificial Insemination:** This is the most popular biotechnological tool easily implemented almost all over India, which ease the job of grading up of the non-descript breed with elite sire. Presently, semen sexing is considered to be one of the best methods to enhance either male or female elite germplasm as per our desire for conservation and genetic improvement.
- **Oestrus Synchronization:** In oestrus synchronization, the manipulation of the bovine oestrus cycle results in standing oestrus in the majority of animals within a short period of time. It is very effective in order to increase the proportion of animals, which are bred at a particular breeding season. Synchronization allows increased use of artificial insemination with the use of elite sires having superior genetic makeup. This technique should be implemented such a way that permissible inbreeding limit (<5 %) should be taken care.
- **Multiple Ovulation and Embryo Transfer (MOET):** In India, very intensive research is going on in embryo biotechnology field, which has resulted in evolving and fine tuning of several embryo related technologies aiming at the multiplication of superior germplasm. Using the standardized protocol for superovulation and embryo transfer, it has been made possible to produce more than 10 calves from a single cow in one calendar year. The objective of this programme is to set up a few elite herds of males and females and carry out the intensive selection and testing within herd/s selecting males and females at an early age using family information. As the genetic merit of males is judged on the basis of performance of their sisters and half-sisters, called as sibling test, not on the performances of their progenies, the generation interval is considerably reduced. Mass MOET with ONBS (Open Nucleus Breeding System) will enable to take care accuracy of selection and faster genetic improvement under field conditions.

Table 1: Breed-wise population growth patterns in indigenous cattle

Breed name	Breeding tract	Census 2007	Breed wise survey 2013			Growth Rate %/annum
			Pure	Graded	Total	
Milch purpose breeds						
Gir	Gujarat (Junagarh, Bhavnagar, Amreli)	21,03,307	13,80,208	37,32,786	51,12,994	28.61
Rathi	Rajasthan (Bikaner, Jaisalmer & Ganganagar)	9,24,087	865921	371588	1237509	6.78
Red Sindhi	Pakistan (Karachi and Hyderabad)	5,49,432	59642	497744	557386	0.29
Sahiwal	Pakistan (Sahiwal District), Ferozpur and Amritsar of Punjab	4,57,405	1090459	3789835	488294	1.35
Dual purpose breeds						
Deoni	Maharashtra (Marathwada region) adjoining parts of Karnataka & AP	1,66,025	151236	200364	383824	26.24
Hariana	Haryana (Rohtak, Hissar, Jind distt) Rajasthan (Alwar, Bharatpur)	26,00,122	1639181	46,40,782	62,79,963	28.31
Kankrej	Gujarat (Kutch, Mehsana, Ahmedabad, Kaira, Sabarkantha), Rajasthan (Barmer, Jodhpur)	38,87,152	1945094	1083185	3028279	-4.42
Krishna Valley	Karnataka (Belgam, Raichur, Bijapur) Maharashtra (Satara, Sangli, Solapur)	2,314	3462	10919	14381	104.30
Mewati	Rajasthan (Alwar, Bharatpur), Uttar Pradesh (Kosi, Mathura)	75,427	14773	18167	32940	-11.27
Ongole	Andhra Pradesh (Chittoor, Kurnool)	2,58,240	115905	518621	634526	29.14
Tharparker	Rajasthan (Jodhpur, Barmer, Jaisalmer)	5,57,679	197291	535182	732473	6.27
Draught breeds						
Amritmahal	Karnataka (Hassan, Chikmaglur, Chitradurga)	98,169	105343	123720	229063	26.67
Bargur	Tamil Nadu (Erode)	21,312	14154	2153	16307	-4.70
Bachaur	Bihar (Sitamarhi, Madhubani, Darbhanga)	4,51,659	741432	805056	1546488	48.48
Binjharpuri	Odisha (Jajpur Subdivision, Cuttack)	46,680	79428	31129	110557	27.37
Dangi	Maharashtra (Nasik, Ahmednagar)	3,04,238	119373	74407	193780	-7.26
Hallikar	Karnataka	21,96,698	1211242	596690	1807932	-3.54
Kangayam	Tamil Nadu (Erode Distt)	3,16,114	80620	112825	193445	-7.76
Khillari	Maharashtra (Solapur, Sangli, Satara)	14,23,742	1102359	911993	2014352	8.30
Malvi	Madhya Pradesh (Dewas, Ujjain, Sajapur distt), Rajasthan (Jhalawar)	15,18,452	1158172	552293	1710465	2.53
Red Kandhari	Maharashtra (Nanded)	1,78,758	235058	222982	458040	31.25
Umblacheery	Tamil Nadu (Thanjavur, Nagapattinam)	2,18,315	39050	33460	72510	-13.36
Dwarf breed						
Vechur	Kerala (Vaikam, Kottayam)	3,170	1065	1414	2479	-4.36
Punganur	Andhra Pradesh (Chittoor)	771	2772	56	2828	53.36

Table 2: Breed-wise population growth patterns in buffaloes

Breed name	Breeding tract	Census, 2007	Breed-wise survey, 2013			Growth rate/annum
			Pure	Graded	Total	
Murrah	Haryana (Rohtak, Hissar)	20,488,438	11686198	36568676	48254874	27.11
Nili Ravi	Punjab (Ferozepur)	591,659	129411	547834	677245	2.89
Bhadawari	Uttar Pradesh (Agra, Etawah), Madhya Pradesh (Bhind, Gwalior)	729,013	583599	1170188	1753787	28.11
Jaffarabadi	Gujarat (Amreli, Junagarh, Bhavnagar)	1,843,848	570177	1200421	1771498	-0.79
Marathwada	Maharashtra (Marathwada region)	183,238	278502	98903	376595	21.10
Mehsana	Gujarat (Mehsana, Ahmedabad)	3,376,196	2676699	948426	3625125	1.47
Nagpuri	Maharashtra (Vidarbha region)	142,765	73584	117410	190994	6.76
Phandharpuri	Maharashtra (Kohlapur, Sangli, Solapur)	272,802	287751	195987	483738	15.46
Surti	Gujarat (Kheda, Vadodra, Bharuch)	2,988,245	1886280	2006614	3892894	6.05
Toda	Tamil Nadu (Nilgiris, Udamanglam, Coonoor distt)	5475	3003	2533	5536	0.22
Banni	Gujarat (Kutch)	527,576	239572	142550	382122	-5.51
Chilika	Odisha	NA	2599	787	3386	NA
Kalahandi	Odisha	NA	115213	26802	142015	NA

References

Das, D.N. (2004). Conservation and propagation of yak genetic resources in India; its problems and prospects. Paper presented at National Symposium on Conservation and Propagation of Livestock and Poultry held on 26-28 February, 2004 at G.B. Pant University of Agriculture & Technology, Pantnagar, Uttaranchal (India).

Guidelines for Management of Animal Genetic Resources, NBAGR, 2016.

Healy, A.A., House, J.K., Thomson, P.C. (2013). Artificial insemination field data on the use of sexed and conventional semen in nulliparous Holstein heifers.J Dairy Sci. pii: S0022-0302(13)00056-8

Nicholas, F.W. (1997). Genetic improvement through technology, Animal Reproduction Science 42: 205-214.

Van Vleck, D. (1981). Prenatal genetic impact of artificial insemination, sex selection, embryo transfer, cloning and selfing in dairy cattle. In: New Technologies in Animal Breeding (B. Brackett, G. Seidel Jr., and S. Seidel). Academic Press, New York. 221-242.

Villanueva, B., Simm, B., and Woolliams, J.A. (1995). Genetic progress and in-breeding for alternative nucleus breeding schemes for beef cattle. Anim. Sci. 61: 231-239.

Wall R.J. (1997). Transgenic livestock: progress and prospects for the future. Theriogenology, 45(1): 57.

□□□

Chapter 6

Breeding Strategies and Programmes for Development of Indigenous Breeds of Cattle and Buffaloes

Kamlesh R. Trivedi, Nilesh Nayee and D.G. Raghupathy

Introduction

Cattle and buffaloes have been an integral part of Indian rural households from time immemorial and playing a critical role in supporting and sustaining livelihoods of a large number of poor. They make large contributions, both in terms of market and non-market services, which include milk, draft power, manure, hides, asset storage, ceremonial services, etc., of the total 147 million rural households, more than 70 million households own at least one cow or buffalo and dairying provides them with a major source of livelihood. About 85% of dairy farmers are small and marginal farmers owning one to three animals. Cattle and buffaloes also provide an equal opportunity for women to participate in decision-making at the household level, as most of the dairy-related activities are done by women. Milk is an important part of food and nutrition security for a largely vegetarian society of 1.2 billion people.

India is considered to be a reservoir of excellent and diverse cattle and buffalo breeds, suited to many diverse agro-climatic conditions. Centuries of natural and human selection have resulted in many genetically diverse breeds fitting into a wide range of environmental conditions, each characterized by its unique adaptive and productive traits. Some of these breeds have acquired characteristics, such as resistance to diseases, resilience to climatic stress, ability to cope with variable access to nutrients, the characteristics that have been lost in some of the high-input exotic breeds due to many years of their selection for one or two productive traits like milk yield, growth, etc. High yielding exotic breeds perform well under optimal environmental, feeding and management conditions, but fail miserably under sub-optimal conditions.

Under an unpredictable future, maintaining genetic diversity allows farmers to choose breeds in response to change in environment, the threat of diseases, changes in feed and water supplies, etc. The loss in genetic diversity erodes their ability to respond to changing conditions. And once genetic diversity is lost, it is lost for ever. Some characteristics of local breeds, which have no commercial value to-day, may become important in the future. Consumers' preferences may change and what is not important today may become important in the future. Genetic diversity, hence, retains the capacity of people to respond to changing consumers' preferences. Some indigenous breeds that survive in extreme environments, such as deserts or other uncultivable lands, provide livelihood to many farmers in such marginal areas. If such breeds are lost, they would take away the main means of their survival.

Presently, these locally adapted cattle breeds are under different levels of endangerment. The last livestock census (2012) observed that the number of indigenous cattle declined by 0.21 per cent annually between 1992 and 2012, whereas that of crossbred cattle increased annually by 6.16 per cent during the same period. This means local cattle have been replaced by crossbreds quite rapidly. In some progressive states like Punjab, the indigenous cow population is nearby zero levels. Crossbred cattle populations have generally been increasing in all states. Though at the country level, the adult female buffalo population has been increasing (increased by 1.29 per cent between 1992 and 2012), in some states, the buffalo population has been declining at an alarming rate particularly in Kerala, Karnataka and Tamil Nadu.

The question then arises is why the number of indigenous cows has been declining and that of crossbred cows increasing. The main factor that drives this change is that farmers get better income from crossbred cows particularly in better resource areas with markets for milk. It is obvious, therefore, that in better resource areas, unless local breeds provide better income than crossbred cows, they will gradually be replaced by crossbreds.

The second question then is: Are there any local breeds that can compete with crossbred cows in favourable resource and market conditions? The answer is yes; some among the indigenous dairy breeds of cattle and buffalo have indeed the scope and potential for development into economically viable animals for livelihood support provided appropriate long-term selection programmes for achieving a steady genetic progress in these breeds are developed in the field, while some others have none, particularly the draft breeds.

This chapter describes the existing genetic resources of local cattle and buffaloes, the efforts that have been made in the field in achieving genetic progress in some of the promising dairy breeds of cattle and buffaloes, the issues to be addressed to achieve a steady and sustained genetic progress in the promising dairy breeds of cattle and buffaloes, and the challenges to be met in maintaining and improving many draft breeds of cattle.

Breeds of Cattle and Buffaloes

The country has a very large population of cattle and buffaloes having many breeds, but their productivity is very low. According to the Livestock Census, 2012, the country had 76.7 million adult female cattle and 56.6 million adult female buffaloes. Out of 76.6 million adult female cattle, 55.4 million (or 72.2%) were indigenous cattle and 21.3 million (or 27.8%) crossbred and exotic cattle (See Table 1). According to the Breed Survey, carried out by DADF, GoI, of the total 55.4 million adult female indigenous cattle, 15.1 million (or 27.2%) were of well-defined breeds and the other 40.3 million (or 72.8%) were non-descript. Similarly, of the total 56.6 million female adult buffaloes, 32.2 million (or 56.9%) were of well-defined breeds and the remaining 24.4 million (or 43.1%) non-descript. The average productivity of in milk indigenous cattle, crossbred cattle and buffaloes per day in 2012 were estimated to be 2.36 kg, 7.02 kg and 4.8 kg, respectively. The average milk yield per day of both local cows and buffaloes had been steadily increasing, whereas that of the crossbreds had been almost constant.

There are 43 well-defined cattle breeds and 16 well-defined buffalo breeds. Of the 41 cattle breeds, 4 are considered as dairy breeds, another 10 as dual-purpose breeds (milk and draft) and the remaining 27 as draft breeds. All buffalo breeds are classified as dairy breeds (See Table 2). Of the total well-defined breeds, the four dairy cattle breeds constitute 32.9 per cent of the total adult female cattle population, 10 dual purpose breeds 31.6 per cent and the 27 draft breeds 35.5 per cent. Overall pure and graded percentages for the cattle breeds were 47 per cent and 53 per cent, respectively and that for buffalo breeds 30 per cent and 70 per cent, respectively. As regards the adult males, in case of cattle they comprise of 30.5 per cent of the total cattle population, whereas in the case of buffaloes, they constitute just 5 per cent of the total buffalo population. This explains that farmers prefer cattle adult males for draft purposes over that of buffaloes. Further, in the case of adult cattle males, adult males of draft breeds are preferred over that of dairy breeds.

Table 1: Population of cattle and buffaloes

Figures are in million

	Cattle					Buffaloes		
	Indigenous Cattle			Exotic & Crossbred	Total cattle	Well-defined breeds	Non-descript	Total
	Well-defined breeds	Non-descript	Total					
Adult Female:								
Pure	7.1 (47.0%)					09.6 (30%)		
Graded	8.0 (53.0%)					22.6 (70%)		
Total	15.1 (27.2%)	40.3 (72.8%)	55.4 (100%) (72.2%)	21.3 (27.8%)	76.7 (100%)	32.2 (56.9%)	24.4 (43.1%)	56.6 (100%)
Female calves	5.0	13.0	18.0	7.0	25.0	11.6	8.5	20.1
Heifers	5.0	11.4	16.4	5.5	21.9	9.5	6.4	15.9
Male calves	3.7	11.4	15.1	3.8	18.9	6.2	4.6	10.8
Adult males	9.1	37.1	46.2	2.1	48.3	2.1	3.2	5.3
Total	37.9	113.2	151.1	39.7	190.8	61.6	47.1	108.7

Source: Breed survey, 2013, DADF, GoI

Table 2: Breeds of cattle and buffaloes

	Adult Females		Adult Males			Adult Females		Adult Males	
	Pop. In '000	% to total	Pop. In '000	% to total		Pop. In '000	% to total	Pop. In '000	% to total
Dairy Breeds					**Buffalo Breeds**				
Gir	2,033	13.5	963	9.9	Murrah	24,928	77.5	1680	81.0
Sahiwal	2,088	13.8	722	7.5	Mehsana	2,002	6.2	50	2.4
Red Sindhi	210	1.4	137	1.4	Surti	2,054	6.4	109	5.3
Rathi	634	4.2	67	0.7	Jaffarabadi	1,038	3.2	33	1.6
Sub total	4,965	32.9	1,889	19.5	Banni	215	0.7	9	0.4
Dual Purpose					Pandharpuri	291	0.9	7	0.3
Kankrej	1,339	8.86	655	6.8	Nagpuri	107	0.3	11	0.6
Haryana	2,668	17.7	1,283	13.3	Bhadawari	892	2.8	92	4.5
Tharparkar	364	2.4	69	0.7	Nili Ravi	370	1.2	19	0.9
Ongole	169	1.1	283	2.9	Toda	2	0.01	0	0
Mewati	15	0.1	6	0.06	Chilka	1.5	0.0	0	0
Krish. Velley	5	0.04	3	0.04	Kalahandi	45	0.1	58	2.8
Deoni	110	0.7	143	1.5	Marathwadi	217	0.7	3	0.2
Gaolao	94	0.6	140	1.5					
Siri	6	0.04	4	0.04					
Sub total	4,771	31.6	2,587	26.7					100
Draft Breeds[1]	5,375	35.6	5,200	53.7					
Breed Total	15,111	27.7	9,676	20.7	Breed Total	32,166	56.8	2,074	39.1
Non-descript	40,306	72.7	37,067	79.3	Non-descript	24,420	43.2	3,224	60.9
Total Ind.	55,417	100.0	46,743	100.0	Total	56,586	100.	5,298	100.

Source: Breed survey, 2013, DADF, GoI; [1]There are 24 draft breeds –Nagori, Kenkatha, Ponwar, Kherigarh, Malvi, Nimari, Red Kandhari, Khillar, Dangi, Amrithmahal, Hallikar, M Gidda, Kangayam, Bargur, Umblachery, Pulikulam, Bachur, Panganur, Kosali, Vechur, Ghumusari, Binjiharpuri, Khariar and Motu.

Genetic improvement programmes for cattle and buffalo breeds in the field

Components of genetic improvement programmes

As a genetic improvement, although additive, is a slow process, any breed improvement programmes need to be considered in the light of requirements of some years ahead. In designing breeding programmes, therefore, it is important to assess the future needs of animals and farmers. Besides, the efforts of conservation and development of indigenous breeds need to be focused in their respective native tract involving a large number of farmers and should lead to making the breed economically relevant to them.

The genetic improvement of any breed of cattle or buffaloes involves the following steps:

i) Defining a breeding goal for breed development - identifying traits that farmers would like to improve and giving weightage to each identified trait;

ii) Developing an appropriate breeding structure for finding the best animals - developing an appropriate infrastructure to record the selected traits and identify those animals that have the highest breeding values for the traits included in the breeding goal;

iii) Dissemination of superior genotype - developing an infrastructure to use the identified best animals to disseminate their superior genotype in the maximum number of animals in the target population;

iv) Building information network to capture data and disseminate information to all stakeholders; and

v) Putting in place systems of quality control for genetic evaluation semen production, AI delivery and information systems.

Defining breeding goals involves collecting information on existing levels of performance on different traits, identifying traits that farmers would like to improve and assigning a goal value to each identified trait. While defining a breeding goal for indigenous breeds of cattle, one has to be very clear on what farmers look for in a breed: Is it milk yield, fat yield, draftability, longevity, disease resistance or combination of these traits with different weightage to each trait?

Having defined a breeding goal for a breed, the next step is to develop an appropriate infrastructure to record the selected traits and identify those animals that have the highest breeding values for the traits, included in the breeding goal.

The type of breeding programme that one can develop and the rate of genetic progress that one can achieve in a target population, primarily depends on the extent of AI infrastructure available in the target population. If a sufficient number of animals are artificially inseminated, progeny testing is a practical and the best option for achieving genetic progress in any population. If AI coverage is inadequate, a breeding structure based on pedigree selection could be considered. In progeny testing, bulls are selected on the basis of their daughters' performance in the field. Since very high selection intensity can be applied on selection of sires and dams to produce the next generation of sires, and very high accuracy in selection of sires could be ensured with the production of a very large number of daughters of bulls, the genetic progress achieved under reasonably large progeny testing programmes is always much higher than other programmes.

In pedigree selection, bulls are selected on the basis of their mothers' and sires' records and bull mothers are selected on the basis of their own records and their mothers' and sires' records. Many different programmes could be developed, depending on the level of AI infrastructure available; for example, a two-tier structure with a nucleus herd and the base population, three-tier structure with a nucleus herd, multiplier herds and the base population, two-tier structure with multiplier herds and the base population.

Having produced the best quality bulls, they need to be used maximally. To maximize the use of best bulls, semen production and processing infrastructure needs to be created to ensure that only the very best bulls produced through genetic improvement programmes are used for semen production and that the semen production and processing technologies are refined to produce an increasing number of doses per bull with high fertilization capacity and no disease-causing organisms. Once quality semen doses are produced using top quality bulls, they need to be carried to farmers' door-step to inseminate their animals. As AI coverage expands in any area, better quality genetics gets disseminated enhancing genetic progress in the population. Two areas need to be focused to provide effective AI delivery services in any area: one, building liquid nitrogen (LN) and semen procurement and delivery system, and second, carrying out inseminations by trained AI technicians with quality semen without harming inseminated animals. Building an information network for capturing data at the source, storing and processing data on a central computer, and generating and disseminating relevant information to all stakeholders is the key factor in successful implementation of any genetic improvement programme.

And finally, to maintain the quality of implementation of the breeding programme, it is important to set minimum standards, put in place an evaluation mechanism and certify bulls that are used for semen production or natural service, semen stations that produce and process semen doses and AI service providers, who provide AI services.

Efforts made in putting genetic improvement programmes in the field

Most of the efforts made in the country for the genetic improvement of indigenous cattle and buffaloes breeds have been primarily restricted to institutional herds. Central Institute for Research on Cattle (CIRC), Meerut has been implementing AICRP (All India Co-ordinated Research Project) on indigenous cattle for important indigenous cattle breeds viz. Gir, Kankrej, Ongole, and Sahiwal through associated herds in collaboration with various veterinary universities, state governments and NGOs (www.circ.org.in, R.S. Gandhi *et al.*, 2013) and supplying quality bulls of indigenous breeds for breeding. There are more than 4000 Gaushalas, which keep a variety of breeds of indigenous cattle; they also contribute to the development of indigenous breeds. The efforts made for the genetic improvement of indigenous breeds of cattle and buffaloes in the field are scanty. National Dairy Development Board has been implementing genetic improvement programmes and more extensively under their National Dairy Plan I (NDP I) beginning 2012. A brief review of progress made for the genetic improvement of indigenous cattle and buffalo breeds Under NDP I is provided in the next section.

Efforts made by NDDB for genetic improvement of indigenous cattle and buffalo breeds

In 1987, NDDB initiated a field progeny testing programme in Mehsana buffaloes in collaboration with Mehsana Milk Union; later in 1992, a similar progeny testing programme for up-graded Murrah buffaloes was commenced in collaboration with Sabarmati Ashram Gaushala and four milk unions, namely Sabar, Panchmahals, Surat and Baroda. In 2003, a pedigree selection programme in the field, each for Kankrej breed in Banaskantha district in Gujarat and for Rathi breed in Bikaner and Shri Ganganagar districts in Rajasthan were initiated.

Once NDP I was launched in 2012, four progeny testing programmes for buffaloes, three for Murrah and one for Mehsana buffaloes and seven pedigree selection programmes, four for cattle breeds, namely Gir, Sahiwal, Hariana and Tharparkar and three for buffalo breeds, namely Jaffarabadi, Nili Ravi and Pandharpuri were added. Both pedigree selection and progeny testing programmes are implemented through following uniform standard operating procedures (SOP) and managed and evaluated through common management and evaluation procedures developed for respective programmes. Data of all events that occur in the projects are collected through a common information system - Information Network for Animal Productivity and Health (INAPH). SOP and monitoring mechanism, followed under pedigree and progeny testing programmes are briefly described below (For details visit NDDB site: www.nddb.org).

SOP for Pedigree Selection Programmes: The project targets native breeding tract of indigenous cattle and buffalo breed. Based on the available secondary information and through a survey, about 50-150 villages with relatively high producing animals of the selected breed are selected as multiplier villages. An infrastructure for artificial insemination is established in multiplier villages and AI services are initiated. All female animals that are inseminated through the project are identified with ear tags, all events of artificial insemination, pregnancy diagnosis and calving of dams are recorded and data entered through INAPH. All high producing animals are put under a systematic milk recording programme. Arrangements are made for inseminating these animals with selected high genetic merit bulls. Farmers are encouraged to rear the male calves born to the elite animals. Male calves are identified with an ear tag and registered in the system as soon as possible. On weaning, calves born to top elite cows are purchased from villagers after parentage testing and disease screening. The purchased males are kept in quarrantine, tested for contagious diseases repeatedly, and are reared in a separate rearing farm after completion of quarrantine. Once matured, the selected bull calves are distributed to semen stations. The semen of very best bulls are used in the multiplier villages of the respective breed, the next best in the base population of the breed in the native tract and the rest for inseminating animals of the respective breed outside the native tract.

Each project is governed by an independent Management Committee represented by all stakeholders and implemented by an independent project team. The project is periodically evaluated by an independent NDDB's evaluation teams.

SOP for Progeny Testing Programmes: A project area covering 100-400 villages in the native tract of the breed with well-developed AI network enabling to carry out minimum 40,000 to 80,000 inseminations is selected. A minimum of 20 bulls of a breed is put to test in the first year and raised to 40 within five years. A minimum of 2000 test doses per bull are distributed in project villages for test inseminations and about 3000 doses per bull are stored till progeny test results of the bulls put to test are available. All female animals that are inseminated with test doses are identified with ear tags. All events of artificial insemination, pregnancy diagnosis and calving of dams are recorded through the INAPH application. All daughters born are identified with ear tags and followed up for growth. When daughters reach serviceable age, they are inseminated with semen from test bulls of future batches and later followed up for pregnancy and calving, all data are recorded through INAPH. Milk production and milk components like fat, protein, lactose, etc. of all the daughters that calves are recorded once a month for a complete lactation. Breeding values of bulls put under test and the milk recorded cows are estimated using a random regression model using test day records. Top 10% of recorded cows/buffaloes based on breeding value are declared as elite animals. The stored semen doses of top 5-10 progeny tested bulls are used for nominated mating of elite cows/buffaloes to produce the next generation of superior bull calves. The bull calves produced through nominated mating are procured after a preliminary selection and subject to meeting the standard protocols of parentage, health, and fitness. After following standard quarrantine and rearing practices, mature bulls are supplied to semen stations.

Each project is governed by an independent Management Committee, represented by all stakeholders and implemented by an independent project team. The project is periodically evaluated by an independent NDDB's evaluation teams.

Progress made so far

The number of villages covered and the number of AI and milk recording centres, established under nine PS projects and six PT projects are given in Table 3.

Table 3: Infrastructure for AI and milk recording under PS and PT projects

Breed	Native districts included	Agency	Project villages	AI centres	Milk recordingc entres
Pedigree Selection Projects:					
Kankrej	Banaskantha	Banas Union	119	50	50
Gir	Bhavnagar, Junagadh	SAG	476	100	100
Rathi	Bikaner, Hanumangarh, Shri Ganganagar	URMUL	201	51	51
Tharparkar	Jaisalmer, Jodhpur, Barmer	RLDB	411	51	51
Sahiwal	Hanumangarh, Shri Ganganagar, Fazilka, Ferozepur, Muktsar, Ludhiana	PLDB and GANGAMUL	330	50	50
Haryana	Sirsa, Fatehabad, Hissar, Jind, Bhiwani, Jhajjar, Rohtak and Sonepat	HLDB	79	39	39
Jaffarabadi	Bhavnagar, Junagadh	SAG	476	100	100
Nili Ravi	Ferozpur, Amritsar, Taran Taran	PLDB	153	50	50
Pandharpuri	Solapur, Sangli	MLDB	156	30	30
Progeny Testing Projects					
Mehsana	Mehsana, Patan, Gandhinagar	Mehsana Union	96	96	96
	Banaskantha	Banas Union	203	75	75
Murrah	Patiala	PLDB	377	133	133
	Jind, Bhiwani, Hissar, Rohtak, Jhajjar, Sonepat	HLDB	297	194	194
	Meerut, Baghpat	ABRO	279	72	72
	Sabarkantha, Panchmahal, Surat, Tapi	SAG	288	147	147

The details of conception rates, service periods, milk yields and fat percentages recorded under different PS and PT projects are given in Table 4. The average conception rate observed in six PS projects of cattle breeds was 45.6%, based on 42,710 recorded AIs and that in three PS projects of buffalo breeds was 37.3%, based on 23,230 recorded AIs. As in PS projects initially, only better-producing animals are put under monthly recording, the average milk yield figures are for the upper segment of the population of each breed. The average 305-day lactation yield and fat% recorded in six cattle PS projects were 2385 kgs. and 4.49%, respectively based on 11,931 observations and that in three buffalo breeds were 2596 kgs. and 7.14%, based on 3020 observations. In six PT projects of buffalo breeds, the average conception rate was 38.4% based on 2,88,973 AIs, the average lactation yield and fat% were 2461 kgs. and 7.4%, respectively based on 41,963 observations. For recently initiated PT projects many selected dams are put under recording, hence the average yield is based on selected dams of different lactations and daughters of the first lactation. The average service periods observed in PS projects of cattle and buffaloes were 139 and 155 days, respectively and that for PT projects of buffalo breeds was 141 days.

Table 4: Details of conception rates, service period and lactation yields recorded under PS and PT projects

Breed	Conception Rate			305-day Lactation Yield			Service Period	
	No. AI	No. PD	CR %	No. Obs.	Avg. yield Kgs. Mean (SD)	Avg. Fat % Mean (SD)	No. obs.	Average in days Mean(SD)
Pedigree Selection Projects:								
Kankrej	7240	3108	42.9	3873	2399(600)	4.3(0.5)	542	134(63.4)
Gir	14222	6068	42.7	1856	2475(693)	5.0(0.8)	249	167(60.6)
Rathi	10945	4921	45.0	2017	2762(522)	3.9(0.4)	407	136(67.7)
Tharparkar	1529	726	47.5	475	2037(404)	-		
Sahiwal -PLDB	866	368	42.5	77	2572(566)	4.2(0.9)		
GANGAMUL	4966	2726	54.9	1023	2295(402)	4.2(0.4)		
Hariana	2942	1574	53.5	2610	2102(422)	4.9(0.8)	52	90(50.4)
Jaffarabadi	14023	5241	37.4	1927	2895(779)	7.5(1.1)	86	172(63.1)
Nili Ravi	5061	1779	35.2	514	2458(558)	6.4(0.7)	10	129(63.1)
Pandharpuri	4146	1649	39.8	579	1722(385)	7.0(0.6)	26	105(37.5)
Total PS - Cattle	42710	19491	45.6	11931	2385	4.49	1250	139
Total-PS Buffalo	23230	8669	37.3	3020	2596	7.14	122	155
Progeny Testing Projects:								
Mehsana-Meh	36253	11040	30.5	7516	1993(511)*	7.4(0.9)	5109	133(70.8)
Mehsana-Banas	25049	10296	41.1	5966	2532(571)	6.8(0.7)	3581	138(69.1)
Murrah-PLDB	51373	20115	39.2	5198	2554(515)	8.0(0.9)	1935	133(66.8)
Murrah-HLDB	87291	35438	40.6	12608	3012(493)	8.0(1.6)	864	123(63.6)
Murrah-ABRO	40564	13181	32.5	1734	2890(653)	6.7(1.1)	919	129(66.1)
Murrah-SAG	48443	20917	43.2	8914	1893(533)*	6.9(1.0)	10167	151(69.8)
Total PT	288973	110987	38.4	41963	2461	7.4	22575	141

Source: INAPH, NDDB as on 30 Oct, 2016, * Records are primarily of daughters in the first lactation

For six PT projects, the details of bulls put to test, bulls completed test mating and production details of daughters of bulls are given in Table 5.

Table 5: Details of bulls testing under six PT buffalo projects

PT Project	Month of starting	Bulls put to test	Bulls completed test	Daughters registered	Daughters complete milk recording	No. of test day records	Avg. 305-days 1st lactation yield in kgs.
Mehsana-Meh	April 87	294	266	44881	6217	59626	1936.3
Mehsana-Banas	Nov 08	96	52	17334	70	650	2193.6
Murrah-PLDB	July 13	86	73	14732	NA	NA	NA
Murrah-HLDB	Feb 14	102	79	8924	NA	NA	NA
Murrah-ABRO	Aug 13	97	69	8038	NA	NA	NA
Murrah-SAG	April 92	327	287	41342	3607	46447	1750.8
Total PT		**685**	**482**	**107531**			

Table 6: Details of estimated breeding values

	305-day Milk Yield				305-day Fat Yield				DPR			
	Mehsana		Murrah		Mehsana		Murrah		Mehsana		Murrah	
TD Rec.	1,091,44		39,593		94,395		18,978		4920		2137	
Avg. TDY	6.34 kg.		6.15 kg.		0.45 kg.		0.42 kg.		37.6		33.2	
Method	RR Animal Model				RR Animal Model				Animal Model			
No. Bulls	247		199		247		195		173		135	
h^2	0.193		0.191		0.101		0.099		0.031		0.071	
Bull Rank	BV	Rel.%	BV	Rel.%	BV	Rel.%	BV	Rel.%	BV	Rel.%	BV	Rel.%
1	410	75	301	84	18	82	12	64	9.01	34	11.72	31
2	403	84	296	75	13	78	8	66	7.78	29	4.86	32
3	369	79	282	79	13	74	7	72	5.39	34	4.71	31
4	335	80	260	79	12	72	4	72	4.13	26	4.02	28
5	325	76	257	73	12	76	4	62	4.13	29	3.94	36
6	305	74	256	76	12	77	4	62	3.61	37	3.13	30
7	302	80	251	78	12	75	4	75	3.59	40	3.08	28
8	294	76	242	81	11	77	2	66	3.48	31	2.65	27
9	290	70	241	85	11	76	0	64	2.68	30	2.44	28
10	279	73	228	84	11	75	0	65	2.56	35	2.15	41

As published on 20 Sept., 2016

❑❑❑

Chapter 7

System Biology Approches in Dairy Cattle Research

T. Saravanan

The emergence of the genome and proteome-enabled platforms have increased our knowledge and understanding of animal biological processes significantly in this era. With the help of systems biology, substantial growth is being witnessed in the various fields of dairy cattle research like nutrition, physiology, breeding, earlier diagnosis of disease and production. For instance, meaningful application of those tools would allow uncovering regulatory checkpoints, which are highly critical during the transition phases of pregnancy to lactation as well as adding nutritional benefits during the growth of young calves. Dietary elements will have the ability to alter gene expression pattern and thus, influence the metabolic profile of dairy and beef cattle. Vast information is already available from the databases generated from whole genome sequencing and transcriptomic profiling of ruminants. Clinical utility of bioinformatic tools are still under validation process and it is time consuming due to the complexity of these systems in interpreting the molecular information. Addressing the knowledge gap arising between computational approaches interconnecting metabolic network programs with fundamental biological functions and sequential implementation of relevant methods in order to generate valuable phenotypic traits, would be of a practical challenge indeed. Prior assessment of risks and minimizing financial distress associated with the implementation programs might require a well-thought-out plan.

Genomic and proteomic approaches have been widely used in personalized human medicine on regular basis. Clinical benefit of these technologies would have been maximised, when the targets or phenotypic traits are being validated by functional approaches. Mitra Biotech has developed such a potential clinically relevant preclinical humanized platform called CANscript™ (strong patent protection across the countries), which helps in segregation of patients who are predicted to respond (as well as predicted not to respond) to anticancer therapeutics.

Successful application of knowledge generated from multiple functional omics technologies in livestock depends on understanding the complexity of networks interconnected with epigenetics, genetics, transcription, translation, protein transport, post-translation modifications, synthesis of metabolites and functional phenotype. The process might slightly be different, when it comes to various cells and tissues or organs. But it offers the advantage of studying the function of thousands of genes, protein molecules or metabolites much rapidly. Selection and careful design of an array experiment is key to generating meaningful outputs and cost-effective results.

Various systems biology tools used in the human and animal settings are described below:

A. Gene Expression - Microarray Platforms

Application

- Genome-wide gene expression studies
- Low to medium sample throughput
- Pre-designed and custom arrays (including design) available
- Whole genome & Exome sequencing
- Mutational analysis
- Genomic selection

Platforms

1. Affymetrix

Affymetrix is used by hundreds of pharmaceutical and biotechnology companies as well as academic, government and other non-profit research institutes to analyze gene expression and genome organization.

- Covers a wide range of organisms for standard 3' gene expression
- Whole transcript expression analysis is available for Human, Mouse, and Rat

Agilent

Agilent Microarray Solutions are based on an integrated, flexible, open approach.

- Custom array design available - to design an optimised array design suitable for customised expression profiling studies
- Pre-Selection strategy (PSS) for optimised array design for expression profiling
- Budget multiplex arrays for standard expression studies, using human, mouse, rat and model organisms available.

Illumina

The Illumina Beadarray platform offers a highly reproducible, multiplex, efficient and cost-effective option for expression studies.

- Standard Whole-Genome Expression Analysis in a multiplex format for Human, Rat, and Mouse
- Whole Genome Expression DASL assay available for partially degraded Human RNA (e.g. FFPE samples)

It is advised to use Illumina recommended protocols and reagents and utilize comprehensive QCs to ensure efficient and high-quality service. Micro-arrays are then scanned using the Illumina Bead Array Reader, and data extracted and normalised (as required) using the Illumina Genome Studio Software.

2. NimbleGen

NimbleGen Systems is a leading supplier of DNA microarrays. NimbleGen's technology joins the ability to make oligo arrays with high density, extreme flexibility, long isothermal probes, up to 4.2 million features, and diverse multiplex formats (3x720K, 4x72K, 12x135K).

ChIP-Chip (Chromatin Immunoprecipitation on microarrays) enables the following

- Revealing gene regulation by determination of promoter occupancy
- Rapid identification of precise binding sites of specific DNA-binding proteins, such as transcription factors, histones, and polymerases

- Mapping gene regulatory networks
- Extended data analysis available.

CGH (comparative genomic hybridization) enables the following:

- Measures DNA copy number differences between a test and reference genome
- Unbiased, genome-wide detection of CNVs down to ~1.4 - 5 Kb resolution
- Rapid prototyping of custom array designs, which can include whole genomes, single chromosomal regions, or multiple loci of interest.

Complete DNA Methylation analysis service enables the following:

- Monitoring of methylation events within the genome
- Comparing differential methylation pattern in cells, tissues or tumour samples
- Extended data analysis available.

B. Proteomic tools

With protein arrays, it will be possible to screen thousands of proteins simultaneously, just as it is for micro-arrays. Protein arrays could be used for many different things, such as detecting presence or absence of proteins, investigating protein expression levels, determining interaction and functions for speciûc proteins, or to look at protein-interactions, protein-protein, protein-antibody or protein-drug.

Phosphoproteomic Array: The PathScan RTK Signalling Antibody Array Kit (Chemiluminescent Readout) is a slide-based antibody array founded upon the sandwich immunoassay principle. The array kit allows for the simultaneous detection of 28 receptor tyrosine kinases and 11 important signalling nodes, when phosphorylated at tyrosine or other residues. Target-specific capture antibodies, biotinylated protein (positive control) and non-specific IgG (negative control) have been spotted in duplicate onto nitrocellulose-coated glass slides.

Integration of knowledge in animal welfare

Integration of knowledge gained from the fields of epigenomics, genomics, proteomics, and metabolomics is a crucial step in the decision-making process and is having an essential role in underpinning the complexity of biological systems toward bio-monitoring animal health, production, reproduction and immunology. Identification of clinically relevant biomarkers led to empowering superior quality systems in farm animal management and offer greater surveillance tools in animal well-being, such as fertility, nutrition, feeding, environmental interaction, health, and disease.

References

Bourneuf *et al.* (2017). Rapid Discovery of De Novo Deleterious Mutations in Cattle Enhances the Value of Livestock as Model Species. Sci Rep. 2017 Sep 13; 7(1): 114-66.

Weber *et al.* (2016). Identification of Gene Networks for Residual Feed Intake in Angus Cattle Using Genomic Prediction and RNA-seq. PLoS One. 2016 Mar 28; 11(3).

R.F. Veerkampemail and B. Beerda, Theriogenology, (2007).

S Naidoo *et al.*, South African J Sci. (2005).

Levensteinet *al.*, BMC Bioinformatics, (2003).

Hanash. Disease Proteomics. Nature, (2003).

Blume-Jensen, P. and Hunter, T. (2001) Nature 411: 355-65.

Graham *et al.* (2010). Affymetrix Human Gene chip array ovine transcriptome UK. Animal Consortium.

Eggen. (2012). The development and application of genomic selection as a new breeding paradigm. Animal Frontiers.

Majumder *et al.* (2015). Predicting clinical response to anticancer drugs using an *ex vivo* platform that captures tumour heterogeneity. Nat Commun. 2015 Feb 27; 6: 61-69.

Gary Hardiman. Pharmacogenomics, (2004).

Schlessinger, J. (2000). Cell 103: 211-25.

Brijwani *et al.* (2017). Rationally, co-targeting divergent pathways in KRAS wild-type colorectal cancers by CANscript technology reveals tumour dependence on Notch and Erbb2. Sci Rep. 4 May, 2017, 7(1): 1502.

□□□

Chapter 8

Conservation of Biodiversity: The Way Forward

S.N. Hegde

The term 'Biological Diversity' was first coined by a wildlife scientist – conservationist, Raymond F. Dasmann in 1968 and was later shortened as Biodiversity by W.G. Rosen in 1985. In the broader version, biodiversity covers the entire life scape of our planet including micro-organisms and is believed to comprise nearly 5.6 million species of the total estimated number of one trillion species. According to the United Nations Environment Programme, biodiversity essentially measures variation at the genetic, species and ecosystem level. Terrestrial biodiversity is rich in the tropics because of warm climate and high primary productivity near the equator. In fact, tropical forests cover about 10% of the earth's surface and harbour around 90% of the known species. Marine biodiversity is denser in the warm coastal waters. Thoughts of conservation biology emerged in the mid-20th century.

Importance of biodiversity as our life-supporting system is rather well-understood. We know that life begets life only if the ambient conditions are favourable for propagation and perpetuation. Causes and effects of biodiversity destruction, such as earthquakes, tsunamis, volcanos, storms, hurricanes, cyclones, floods, and drought are better highlighted than the ways and means of protecting it. Against rising global population and the concomitant array of civilizational needs [for housing, industry, transport, energy, commerce, agriculture, communication, etc], it has been a great challenge to safeguard biodiversity in its totality. The severe climatic change affects both the biological and physical world. For instance, the recent events, such as hurricanes in the U.S. and the Caribbean, monsoon deficiency in India, heat waves in Europe, drought in Australia, flooding in South Asia, melting of Arctic and Antarctic ice, rising sea levels, increasing global temperature (compared to pre-industrial era) and associated phenomena have significantly threatened biodiversity.

Ways and Means of Conservation

The concept of conservation should be a way of life as it has been practised in India by the 'Adivasis', tribals and people, who live in the periphery of forests. We have to bear in mind that our forefathers had left this planet in a 'livable' state and hence, we have the bounden obligation to leave it behind in a comparable (if not similar) condition. We certainly need to come out of the mindset that all natural resources and treasures belong only to our 'present' and nothing is to be preserved/conserved for the 'future'. This is a highly short-sighted, ill-conceived and self-centric attitude. Our basic need is justifiable but not the unbridled greed. Modern society, unfortunately, has become more materialistic and less futuristic. Even increasing consumerism and the desire to raise the standard of living (if not life), have led to overexploitation of natural wealth occurring in the form of biodiversity.

Our country is endowed with rich human, physical and biological resources (more precisely 'reserves' for, reserves are transformed as resources only after value addition). Biological diversity offers genetic diversity, which is the precious product of millions of years of organic evolution tested and retained through Darwin's theory of natural selection and survival of the fittest. It implies that it takes millions of years for a species to evolve and each one is unique from this perspective.

Minimizing the degradation of natural habitats/ecosystems is one of the best ways of protecting biodiversity. But this is easier said than done. It entails considerable planning of our developmental schemes with a high degree of coordinated, integrated and sustainable concepts. Environmental issues warrant multi-pronged action through multi-agencies. Many developing countries including India have not been able to maintain a harmonious synergy between requirements and approaches. This imbalance or mismatch has often threatened our invaluable biodiversity, be it in the Himalayan and Nilgiri Biospheres or the Western Ghats – declared by UNESCO as the 'world heritage site' and considered 'hyper hot' for conservation.

The Centre for Ecological Sciences, IISc, Bangalore has a database of about 5000 species of vascular plants found in the Western Ghats. Of these, the Centre has identified 20 critically endangered, 72 endangered, 24 threatened and 63 species of vulnerable plants. Genetic potential of important wild plants (e.g. with medicinal properties – we have 6500 of them) and animals (e.g. the lion-tailed monkey), if understood properly, could contribute immensely to future research in biotechnology opening new avenues of plant and animal production. Of particular importance is the conservation of our endemic species of plants and animals.

It must be emphasized that the Western world has totally failed to appreciate that there is an ethical approach to conservation. For instance, simple and balanced lifestyles with less demand for fossil fuels, such as coal, oil, and gas, leads to decreased energy consumption. The so-called HDI (human development index) of the UN does not consider the noble values and philosophy of life and living. It was reported that some of the virgin stretches of forests in Asian sub-continent remained so because of religious taboos against tree felling (the so-called religious basis of conservation). In Karnataka, such sites are called 'Devarakadus' and 'Nagarabanas'. We need to explore newer strategies of conservation and adopt new norms (do's and don'ts) say, of slowing down the pace of industrialization (it seems China is practicing this), checking population growth and increased switchover to solar-wind-hydro-bio-sources of clean energy. Decreased global population, if realized, naturally will reduce energy consumption. It is well-known that one of the greatest threats to biodiversity is the human interference of unprecedented scale.

Apart from effective educational programmes through schools, print and electronic media, laws on hunting, poaching, pollution, illegal logging and felling of trees, trade on plants and animal products, mining, etc. must be vigorously enforced with severe punishment [we have greatly failed on this measure]. Ignorance of the law can be pardoned but not wanton disobedience or flouting of the law. In our country, many crimes go either unnoticed or unpunished because of the weakness of law-enforcing authorities.

The tendency to resort to mega projects should be curtailed. There could be smaller units of irrigation and power generation. The routes of new highways and railway lines must be thoughtfully chosen. Eco-auditing or the cost and benefit of large developmental plans (e.g. dams) must be done scientifically with reliable data. The dictum or the guiding principle should be "development – yes, but environmental safeguards–first". Wherever tampering is inevitable (e.g. mining and widening of roads), efforts must be made to re-store and rejuvenate the ecosystems. This was done successfully in many other countries, especially upon large scale mining operations. Conservation warrants fewer slogans and more actions.

Application of new technologies

Science gives rise to technologies that can act as double-edged swords. Application of technologies could be destructive as well as productive. In terms of conservation of biodiversity (say of rare endemic and endangered species of plants and animals), we have new techniques of tissue culture (micro-propagation), cryopreservation of semen, eggs and embryos and their long-distance transportation by air, cloning, translocation, captive breeding, superovulation, IVF, embryo transfer, surrogacy and production of transgenic plants and animals. Well-protected national parks, wildlife reserves (reserve forests), sanctuaries, safaris, zoological and botanical parks, massive aforestation, rejuvenation of rivers, lakes and wetlands - all will enhance biodiversity conservation.

Apart from the government schemes, it must be reiterated that people's involvement at the grassroots level, as partners in conservation of biodiversity, is of paramount importance. Without citizens', participation and co-operation, we cannot safeguard our landscape as wells as lifescape. Finally, our teaching institutions at primary, secondary and tertiary levels should expose the students to the marvels of biodiversity for ensuring human welfare through proper climate, health, and food security. Notwithstanding the catastrophe of the kind of Jurassic Period, the future of mankind is inextricably linked with the abundance of biodiversity.

References

Gaston, Kevin, J. (2000). Global patterns in biodiversity. Nature, 405: 220-227.

Field, Richard and 12 others, (2008). Spatial species-richness gradients across scales: a meta-analysis J. Biogeography, 36: 132-147.

Soule, Michael E. (1986). What is conservation biology? Bioscience, 35: 729-734.

Davis Peter, (1996). Museums and the natural environment: the role of natural history museums in biological conservation. Leicester University Press.

Dyke, Fred Van, (2008). Conservation Biology: Foundations, concepts, applications. Springer Science & Business Media.

❑❑❑

Chapter 9

Gaushala as a Focal Point for Conservation of Indigenous Cattle Genetic Resources

D.K. Sadana

Introduction

Indigenous cattle genetic resources are the 43 hitherto registered breeds in the country (e.g. Gir, Tharparkar) along with the 29 'lesser-known breeds' of cattle (e.g. Nari, Alambadi), and the third group that are unique populations that have been noticed but not studied in detail (e.g. Umarda of Maharashtra, Malaimadu of Tamil Nadu). The registered breeds (first group) are well-documented and cover some 20% of the total cattle population in the country; the lesser known breeds (the second group) are also termed as 'defined but yet not registered populations' should be around 10% of the total indigenous. The remaining 70% indigenous population, often classified as 'non-descript' has several subpopulations in different ecosystems that could be unique and distinct from others. Presently, these are classified within 'non-descript'. Sooner or later, such populations will be identified and described. It can be argued that this third group makes some 10% of the indigenous cattle population. Remaining 60% of indigenous cattle are at present non-descript or a mix-up of other breeds/ populations. In terms of share, indigenous cattle in the country makes 79% while the rest (21%) are exotics and crossbreds [Rashtriya Gokul Mission, GoI, 2017]. Gaushalas in the country (numbering some 4000) are perceived as the locations with large herds of mixed up cattle. Studies, however, have revealed the presence of a good number of purebreds in several Gaushalas. Of all the cattle in the Gaushalas, as many as 22.2% are purebred indigenous cattle (Sadana, 2005). This feature has variously been utilized to develop Gaushalas as conservation centres for the local breeds with some notable success stories in Haryana and Rajasthan. While this challenge is met, a Gaushala can be promoted to act as a focal point for local breed conservation within proximal Gaushalas as well as in surrounding villages within the breed tract.

Cattle Conservation

Conservation is an essential activity to save a population from extinction. Cattle conservation is the management of the given cattle breed in sufficient numbers, preferably in its home tract in a manner that the animals survive and produce and are useful to the present generation while retaining potentials of being useful to future generations as well. Alternately, conservation is raising the number of animals, where these are less than the desired number or in endangered level. There are two basic modes, in which conservation is accomplished. A breed conserved at its own site i.e. in its own habitat and in the same manner, in which the animals are naturally found i.e. with farmers or breeders in villages or their natural systems is termed as *in-situ* conservation. Since the animals are conserved as 'live animals', it is also termed as *in-situ in-vivo* conservation. Animals conserved beyond its natural habitat is termed as *ex-situ* conservation. Under *ex-situ,* the animals can be conserved as live animals e.g. Gir cows of Gujarat taken to Andhra Pradesh and maintained there for a long time. This is termed as *ex-situ in-vivo* conservation. Or, secondly, the animals can be conserved in the form of semen or embryos or cells or DNA fragments under laboratory conditions like cryopreservation, which is termed as *ex-situ in-vitro* conservation. In general, parlance and in practical conditions, however, *in-situ* conservation is the conservation of the breed at the farmers' level and *ex-situ* conservation is the conservation of semen under cryopreservation. The best form of livestock conservation is to raise their numbers in their natural environment since the animals continue to be exposed to the environmental strengths/stresses and continue to evolve and stay in tune with the changing conditions.

Need for Conservation

Local cattle breeds are well-adapted to local conditions - a reduction in their numbers means reduced dependence of local marginal people on local production systems. Local cattle are able to utilize the local bio-mass more effectively. Hence, reduction in numbers also means the locally available bio-mass goes unutilized. Local breeds are more resistant to diseases and scarcely need any medicines. Reduction in their numbers also means we are losing robust systems and replacing with medicine-dependent production systems. All this is beside the loss of Desi cow milk, which is known for being safe A2 type, has a higher percentage of the useful CLA (Conjugated Linoleic Acid), a higher percentage of the beneficial O3Fa (Omega-3-Fatty Acids) and also, a higher percentage of cerebrosides. Reduction in local cattle leads to reduced availability of young bulls for field agricultural work, where these continue to be ineffective use in all the states. The most prominent cause of the reduction in indigenous cattle breeds is the low milk yield of the local breeds in the prominent presence of easy alternatives *i.e.* high yielding crossbreds and mechanical draft power for field operations. Both these 'easy alternates' are under scanner now, in terms of doubtful quality of milk and the ever-spreading pollution due to mechanization. Besides, the quality milk from the indigenous cattle, the emphasis has not been given to several other benefits received viz. cow-dung for organic farming & energy, cow-urine for bio-pesticide & medicinal use, and draft power for pollution-free energy that is renewable. All these reasons suggest that the cattle breeds need to be conserved for being locally adapted systems providing therapeutic nutrition, environmentally-safe energy, soil health and monetary benefits besides being an integral part of the local biodiversity. Thereby, most crucial factors to conserving local cattle breeds, in the present context are: (1) raising milk yield of the cattle breeds, and (2) emphasizing the utility and proper utilization of all the products and clean energy resources from the local breeds.

Indigenous Cattle Genetic Resources

The 43 registered breeds (30 extant and the 15 recently registered since 2010) along with the 25 defined populations (Lesser Known Breeds), and few more locally recognized populations: all these together make the 'Indigenous Cattle Genetic Resources' of the country. Each of these populations is important, as each belongs to its own eco-system and it is well-known that "a breed in its own eco-system is the most efficient production system". The populations in group 2 and group 3 have not been recognized/registered so far only because these have neither been characterized till now, nor the special features of these populations recorded hitherto. There is indeed a need to increase these populations, as these are adapted to local conditions and are easily manageable using traditional knowledge, and these are meeting local requirements like draught power, manure, etc. more effectively. Indigenous cattle breeds and populations have to be discussed vis-à-vis the Gaushalas in the breed tract: a Gaushala in the vicinity can prove to be an important resource to help conserve the local breeds.

Gaushalas in India

Presently, there are more than 4000 Gaushalas in India and most of these act as a shelter for old, unproductive and diseased cows. Although present in almost all the districts in the country, Gaushalas are more prevalent in Gujarat, Haryana, Rajasthan, and Uttar Pradesh. There is a relatively low frequency of Gaushalas in North-Eastern states. Earlier considered as a medium for cattle just to complete the lifespan, studies during the last decade revealed the presence of more local cattle purebreds within Gaushala than the number outside Gaushala. This raised interest in Gaushalas, especially the Gaushalas selected on the basis of the presence of a good number of local purebreds and sufficiently good infrastructure. Several Gaushalas in the country have made significant progress in different aspects: some are self-sufficient and do not need donation or support from outside (e.g. Ladwa Gaushala, Hissar, Haryana), some other Gaushalas have excelled in maintaining purebred indigenous breeds in good numbers (e.g. Noor Mahal Gaushala, Nakodar, Punjab), still other Gaushalas have excelled in production and supply of A2 milk (e.g. Bansi Gaushala, Ahmedabad), and some Gaushalas have saved the local breeds (e.g. Varanasi Gaushala saving Gangatiri breed). In several Gaushalas, the management is aware to improve the local cattle breed. These progressive ones and such other Gaushalas have attempted and achieved some level of conservation of the local cattle breed.

Gaushalas as Focal Point for Conservation

In a survey, made during 2004-05 in 59 Gaushalas of North-West India, it was observed that there are some Gaushalas that are carefully maintaining a good number of cattle of one or two local breeds. Of these, 21 Gaushalas were earmarked as potential ones for saving the local breeds, based on sufficient infrastructure facilities and awareness of the management. Such Gaushalas can be developed as focal points for genetic improvement and conservation of indigenous cattle breeds.

As per the existing status in these Gaushalas, it was noted, the purebred animals were interspersed in all the mixed animals and the unselected males also roamed about in the herd leading to further dilution of the purebreds; the progeny was not better than the parents. A new model was developed to circumvent this problem. Named as '10-P Model', it requires separating out the purebreds of given breed animals from the Gaushala herd and keeping these in a separate barn within the Gaushala. A good bull needs to be provided in this barn to expect genetically improved progeny. Over time, young bulls from this barn can be used in the remaining Gaushala for genetic improvement and also, be used in the surrounding villages for overall regional improvement of the breed. Modern practices need to be used in the 10P Barn like sufficient feed/fodder and health support and recording for proper selection and genetic improvement. Gaushala, hence, can be used as a focal point for breed conservation within the Gaushala, in surrounding Gaushalas and in surrounding villages.

Enhanced utilization of all the products from the indigenous cattle providing better incomes to the farmers will further boost local breed conservation. It is important to utilize special features of the local breeds e.g. A2 and therapeutic milk, better quality dung from the local breeds, use of cow urine in the preparation of some medicines and as bio-pesticide for organic and natural farming.

Epilogue

Fuller utilization of all the cow products viz. A2 milk, cow-urine, quality dung, and draught power for improved livelihoods and emphasis to now feasible genetic improvement in the 10P Barn can make selected Gaushalas be the focal point for conservation of local cattle breeds.

□□□

Chapter 10

Novel Reproductive Technologies for Conservation of Animal Genetic Resources

P.S.P. Gupta, S. Nandi and S. Mondal

Long-term preservation of germ cells, embryos, and even the somatic cells would help in the conservation of our valuable animal genetic resources. There are several novel reproductive techniques are available that facilitate the conservation of Animal Genetic Resources like *in vitro* production of embryos (IVP), Oocyte cryopreservation, Embryo cryopreservation, Preantral follicle technology (PFT), Cloning, Somatic cell Nuclear transfer, Stem cell technology, and sperm sexing.

In vitro production of Embryos (IVP)

Oocyte retrieval

Oocytes can either be collected from abattoir-derived ovaries or live animals. Collection of oocytes from live superior animals lead to the production of quality embryos.

Oocyte recovery from live animals

'Ovum pick up (OPU)' or transvaginal oocyte recovery (TVR) using ultrasonography permit the repeated non-surgical collection of oocytes from superior donor cows OPU performed on hormone (FSH, GnRH) stimulated heifers resulted in significantly higher recovery of good quality oocytes and higher blastocyst yield following IVP compared to that performed on unstimulated ones.

In vitro maturation of oocytes

Follicle enclosed oocytes are arrested at the diplotene stage of the prophase of first meiotic division. Maturation of oocytes includes the completion of two cellular programs: (1) Nuclear maturation –

Resumption of meiosis from the germinal vesicle to metaphase II stage and (2) Cytoplasmic maturation: Molecular and structural changes that provide the matured oocytes with the capacity to support fertilization and early embryonic development.

Oocytes are generally cultured in Tissue Culture Medium (TCM)-199 or Ham's F-10 medium and may or may not be supplemented with serum (fetal bovine serum, calf serum, serum from animals at different stages of the estrous cycle, steer serum), hormones (FSH, LH, estradiol 17b, progesterone, prolactin, growth hormone and feeder cells (granulosa cells, oviductal epithelial cells, Vero cells). Oocytes are incubated at 38.5-39.5^0 C for 24 hours in 5% CO_2 in the air to achieve the maturation. Though maturation rate of oocytes are assessed by various methods like staining method (M II stage), degree of cumulus cells expansion and identification of extruded first polar body in the perivitelline space; degree of expansion of cumulus cell mass is routinely employed in buffalo IVM studies for evaluating oocyte maturation for its use in *in vitro* fertilization. Current research aims at mimicking the effects of follicular dominance on 'oocyte capacitation' by blocking nuclear oocyte maturation in order to allow for cytoplasmic capacitation before nuclear maturation is resumed.

In recent times, the costly additives, which are commonly used in IVM medium *i.e.* fetal calf serum, hormones are being replaced effectively by the economical additives like estrous cow serum, steer serum, follicular fluid, cystic follicular fluid, etc. The costly pure FSH is effectively being replaced by the economical PMSG. But the practice of addition of hormones like LH and FSH to the IVM medium is still being followed by many laboratories.

In vitro fertilization of Oocytes (IVF)

In vitro matured oocytes are coincubated with frozen-thawed *in vitro* capacitated spermatozoa in Tyrode's modified medium or Brackett and Oliphant medium for fertilization. The separation of motile cattle and buffalo bull sperm after thawing was achieved by swim up or Percoll gradient technique. High fertilization and cleavage rate have been obtained by using various sperm motility enhancer like heparin, caffeine, glutathione and hypotaurine, theophylline, a mixture of penicillamine, hypotaurine and epinephrine (PHE). Considerable variations were reported among different bulls in terms of the ability of their spermatozoa to fertilize oocytes and blastocyst production *in vitro*. Sperm concentration and prolonged oocyte-sperm co-incubation during *in vitro* gamete interaction reported affecting subsequent embryo development. A sperm dose of 0.25 X 10^6 to 0.5 X 10^6 and 15-20 hours sperm-oocyte co-incubation is found to be optimum for cattle IVF.

In vitro Embryo Culture (IVC)

In most laboratories, blastocyst production *in vitro* is 30-60% and 15-30% of inseminated oocytes, in cattle and buffalo, respectively, in spite of numerous variations of the basic techniques. Three systems of culturing embryos *in vitro* are commonly used. First, cleaved embryos are cultured in the oviduct of sheep (*in vivo* culture,). Second, cleaved embryos are cultured *in vitro* in basic medium (TCM-199, B2, Minimum Essential medium) supplemented with serum and somatic cells (oviductal epithelial cells, cumulus cells, buffalo rat liver cells or in medium conditioned by somatic cells. Somatic cells are reported to secrete proteins, embryotrophic factors (Tissue inhibitor of metalloproteinase-1 (TIMP-1), growth factors and remove inhibitory components from *in vitro* culture environment of the embryo. Third, cleaved embryos are cultured in simple defined media (Thompson, 2000), where components are in accordance with the needs of embryos. Due to variability in composition and risk of infection in complex media, research has been focused on embryo culture using serum-free defined media. The most common defined medium for *in vitro* culture is synthetic oviductal fluid (SOF) or a modified form of SOF. Except for a very few studies, where defined media have been used for culture of buffalo embryos, most investigators used complex media containing serum and somatic cells.

Generation of embryos using novel techniques

In recent times, embryos are being produced by novel techniques i.e. production of embryos using oocytes retrieved from *in vitro* grown preantral follicles, nuclear transfer, embryo splitting/cloning, etc.

Preantral follicle technology (PFT)

Cows are born with thousands of primordial and preantral follicles, of which less than 1% ovulate in the reproductive life. Harvesting oocytes only from antral follicles limit the number of offspring per animal and the optimal exploitation of the genetic material. There is a scope for developing the preantral follicles *in vitro* into antral follicles for IVM and IVF. Bovine primordial and preantral follicles are successfully isolated and cultured. Follicular antrum development has been accomplished recently in cattle by culturing large preantral follicles (166 mm) upto 28 days. Effective isolation and culture protocols for preantral follicles were developed for many of the domestic animals i.e. cattle, buffalo. Embryo production from oocytes derived from *in vitro* grown preantral follicles was reported only for pigs, sheep, and buffalo. The basic steps in this specific technology are only two i.e. Isolation of preantral follicles and *in vitro* culture of preantral follicles. When the preantral follicles grow to the stage of Graafian follicle *in vitro*, the oocyte is isolated and IVF is performed using conventional methods.

Cloning and Somatic Cell Nuclear Transfer Technology

Nuclear transfer (NT) is a relatively efficient technology to produce transgenic animals as well as multiple copies of proven or endangered animals by cloning. Nuclear transfer involves the introduction of the nucleus from a totipotent donor cell into a matured enucleated oocyte. The resulting embryo is transferred to a surrogate mother for development into a live offspring. Key to the overall success of NT is the requirement for totipotency; defined here as the potential to initiate and direct normal development. Although many of the factors controlling totipotency have yet to be elucidated, blastomeres and various cell types from fetal and adult origin have been successfully used to clone a number of different species, including farm animals, such as sheep, goats, and cattle.

General procedure of nuclear transfer technique

Recipient cytoplasts for nucleus transfer are obtained by *in vitro* maturation (IVM) of oocytes. After 20-24 h of maturation culture, cumulus cells of oocytes are removed by repeated pipetting through a fine-bore pipette in BSA-free PB1 containing 1 mg/ml hyaluronidase. Oocytes with the first polar body (metaphase II oocytes) are selected as recipient oocytes. Oocytes are enucleated by aspirating the first polar body and adjacent ooplasm (about 1/3 of an ooplasm) using an enucleation pipette (diam. 35 μm) in PB1 + 20% FCS containing 5 μg/ml CB and 0.1 μg/ml colcemid. Briefly, an oocyte is oriented and fixed in a holding pipette with its first polar body positioned at 3 o'clock.

Enucleation pipette is introduced through the zona pellucida into the perivitelline space, and the first polar body with adjacent cytoplasm that contained a spindle of metaphase II is delicately sucked into the pipette and pulled out from the perivitelline space. To enucleate 25–30 oocytes, it takes 1.5 h. Recently, chemical induced enucleation using certain chemicals like cycloheximide, taxol, and demecolcine was also reported. To confirm the removal of the M II chromosomes, fragments of removed ooplasm are stained with 5 µg/ml acridine orange for 5 min and observed using a fluorescent microscope. Reliability of enucleation is tested usually by Hoechst-staining. We can use Hoechst staining also. After 22 h of maturation culture, enucleated oocytes are activated by electric impulse or by exposure to 7% ethanol in maturation medium for 7 min and further cultured in maturation medium containing 5 µg/ml cycloheximide for 6 h. The same enucleation pipette can be used to aspirate the disaggregated donor cell and place it into the perivitelline space of the enucleated oocyte. Fusion of NT couples is induced by one 15-µsec, 2.0-kV/cm DC pulse in a 3.5-mm fusion chamber (BTX). Fusion medium is generally 0.25 M D-sorbitol containing 0.1 mM calcium acetate, 0.5 mM magnesium acetate, 0.5 mM Hepes, and 1 mg/ml fatty acid-free BSA. Fused NT embryos are IP_3 + DMAP-activated and cultured to the blastocyst stage in EBSS-complete medium.

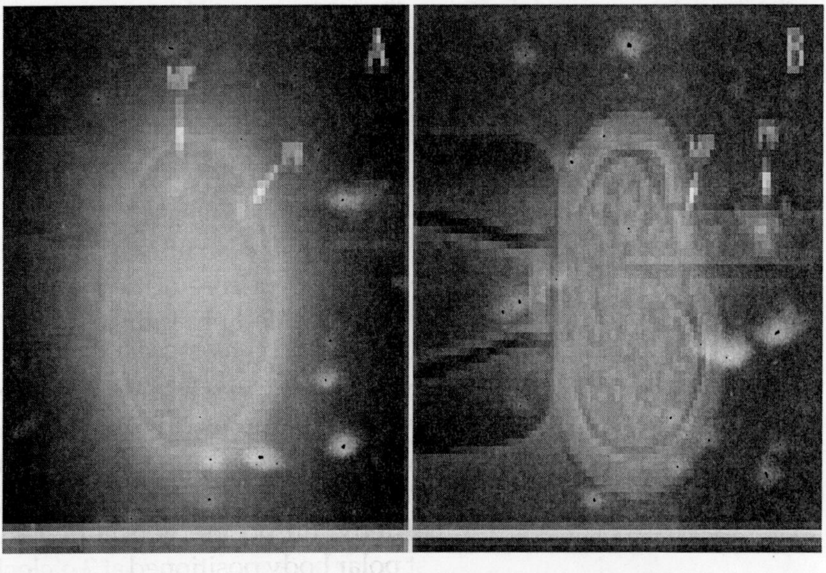

Figure 1: Enucleation of oocyte A. introduction of a microneedle into perivitelline space, B.Aspiration of metaphase plate (MP) and polar body (PB)

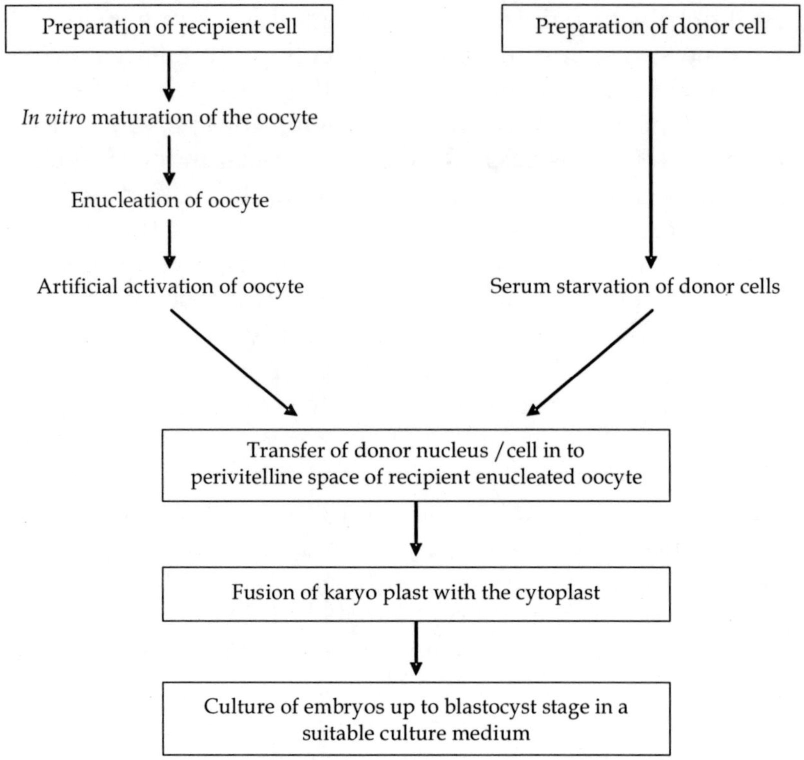

Figure 2: Procedure involved in the production of embryos by nuclear transfer technique

Embryonic stem cells

Embryonic stem cells (ES cells) were established for the first time in mouse, using inner cell mass (ICM) cells from delayed blastocysts cultured in embryonal carcinoma culture medium and from normal blastocysts cultured in embryonal carcinoma culture conditioned medium. ES cells were also established from blastomeres of morulae. Differentiation of the embryonic cells in culture is effectively prevented by feeder layers of the embryonic fibroblast cell line, primary murine embryonic fibroblasts, buffalo rat liver cell conditioned medium in combination with feeder cells, or defined media, containing leukaemia inhibitory factor **(LIF)** but no feeder cells.

Primordial and Embryonic germ cells

Primordial germ cells (PGC) also called fetal germ cells (FGC) are the founder cells of the germ cell line that develop into gametes after meiosis. Embryonic germ cells (EGC) are pluripotent cell lines established from PGC. Since gametes acquire totipotency after fertilization, it is hypothesized that PGC may possess pluripotency or totipotency. If this is true, then PGC or FGC could be good candidates for production of cloned and transgenic offspring. Mouse PGCs supported development to blastocyst stage, when subjected to nuclear transfer or embryo aggregation. It was also reported that PGC from male fetuses supported development to blastocyst stage more frequently than those from female fetuses. EGC were successfully established from PGC in this species. The culture system used for obtaining pluripotent cell lines from PGC, in general, was similar to those used for ES cells. FGC was preserved at 4°C and subsequently, their ability to develop into blastocysts was established.

Sperm sexing

Pre-selection of offspring sex at the time of conception is the most sought-after reproduction techniques of all time. Sperm sexing methods are based on the differential amount of DNA being present in the X and Y-chromosome bearing sperm. Sort analysis of DNA content by flow cytometry, fluorescence *in situ* hybridization (FISH) and use of polymerase chain reaction (PCR) on individual sperm are effective for assessing samples for the proportion of X and Y sperm. At present times, the flow cytometric sorting method and modified high-speed sorting provide the only fully validated means of sperm sexing.

Embryo splitting and sexing

Embryo splitting facilitates induction of twinning, embryo sexing and an increase in the number of transferable embryos. Direct transfer of embryos yielded around 60 calves per 100 embryos; transfer of split embryos typically produced 105 calves per 100 embryos. The sex of the preimplantation embryos can be diagnosed fairly accurately with a variety of procedures and it is used routinely in multiple ovulation embryo transfer (MOET) scheme of embryo transfer in cattle (Wilmut *et al.*, 2000).

Conclusions

Some technologies like preantral follicle development for the embryo resource generation needs further attention since no offspring could be produced till date using this technology in any of the species excepting rodents. Laboratory production of embryos has been standardized for most of the domestic animals and can be used as a successful tool for the embryo resource generation for the conservation of livestock species. Production of embryos using novel techniques like the nuclear transfer is helpful in the production of value-added farm animals. Embryo resources generation using these novel techniques will effectively reduce the generation, interval and helps in effective conservation of germplasm of both indigenous breeds of farm animals and endangered species. Further, research is necessary for successful usage of preantral follicles in the generation of viable embryos. Standardization of techniques of laboratory production of embryos both by normal and nuclear transfer method would lead to the establishment of embryo banks for the conservation of indigenous livestock and endangered species.

References

Gupta, P.S.P. and Nandi, S. (2012). Isolation and culture of preantral follicles for retrieving oocytes for the embryo production: Present status in Domestic Animals. *Reproduction in Domestic Animals* 47: 513-519.

Gupta, P.S.P., Nandi, S., Ravindranatha, B.M. and P.V. Sharma (2001). Isolation of preantral follicles from buffalo ovaries. *Veterinary Record.* 148: 543-544.

Gupta, P.S.P., Nandi, S., Ravindranatha, B.M. and Sharma, P.V. (2002). *In vitro* culture of buffalo (*Bubalus bubalis*) preantral follicles. *Theriogenology* 57: 1839-1854.

Gupta, P.S.P., Nandi, S. and Sharma, P.V. (1999). Augmentation of Reproductive efficiency in ruminants. Technical bulletin No.3. National Institute of Animal Nutrition and Physiology, Bengaluru, India.

Gordon, I. (2005). Laboratory production of cattle embryos. 2nd edition, CABI publishing. Oxford University Press.

Nandi, S., Ravindranatha B.M. Raghu, H.M. and Chauhan, M.S. (2002). Production of buffalo embryos *in vitro*: Premises and Promises. *Reproduction in Domestic Animals* 37: 65-74.

Jiang, J. and Ott, T.L. (2010). Reproductive Genomics in Domestic animals. Wiley-Blackwell Publishers. 1st edition.

□□□

Chapter 11

Ultrasound Guided Ovum Pick-up: A Technology for Oocyte Recovery from Animals for Germplasm Conservation

S. Jeyakumar

Introduction

Efficient exploitation of the female gamete pool and a shortening of the generation interval are the most important aims in modern dairy husbandry. In the early 1970s, Superovulation or Multiple ovulation and Embryo Transfer (MOET) were developed. Embryo transfer technology offers the opportunity for efficient exploitation of the female gamete pool and shortening of generation interval (Hansen and Block, 2004). However, the use of this technology as a tool for enhancing reproductive efficiency is limited by the high cost of producing embryos, the variable and unpredictable superovulatory response of donor cows, the low embryo yield. Following the birth in 1978 of Louise Brown, the first IVF baby, the research efforts into developing similar techniques for the bovines increased, which resulted in 1981 in the birth of Virgil, the first IVF calf (Brackett *et al.*, 1982). The practical application of *in vitro* production of embryos depends on the abundant availability of developmentally competent cumulus-oocyte complexes from valuable donor cows. Aspirating follicles from ovaries of a slaughtered animal is currently the most common procedure, but represents a non-repeatable approach and since the genetic origin of the oocyte is unknown, such oocytes are not of interest to researchers engaged in work for breeding programmes. Alternatively, laparoscopic or endoscopic procedures for follicular aspiration have been used initially for the retrieval of oocytes from the living animal. However, these procedures are either too traumatic and/or not repeatable enough to be effective for routine collection of immature oocytes needed for large scale IVM/IVF/IVC programmes from valuable donors.

Ultrasound-guided transvaginal follicular aspiration (TVFA) combined with *in vitro* maturation, fertilization and culture (IVMFC) emerged as a method for producing pre-implantation stage bovine embryos that are suitable for transfer to establish a pregnancy. This paper will address the major developments in the field of Ovum Pick-up (OPU), procedure, efficiency, future applications and limitations of OPU.

OPU Technology: History and Developments

The technology of OPU/IVP aims at harvesting (immature) oocytes from living animal by ultrasound-guided transvaginal follicular aspiration (USG-TVFA), followed by *in vitro* maturation, fertilization and culture until embryos have reached the morula or blastocyst stage and can be transferred non-surgically into recipients or frozen or used for research at any stage of development.

The major breakthrough occurred in the field of human Assisted Reproductive Technology was when researchers developed Ultrasound-guided transvaginal oocyte aspiration (Gleichert *et al.*, 1983 and Dellenbach *et al.*, 1984) and then the technology was adopted in the bovine in 1987, in Denmark (Callesen *et al.*, 1987). Currently, OPU and IVF considered as a well-adapted and promising technologies in the field of assisted reproductive technology. In addition, with recent developments in genome sequencing and availability of chips for screening/selection of key genes for traits of economic importance becoming available in the recent years, OPU/IVP has proven as invaluable technology for rapid genetic improvement. Brazil dominated the IVP production by performing 53,019 OPU sessions averaging 15 oocytes and 6 embryos per session (Qi *et al.*, 2013). There are many embryo technology companies worldwide including India, who are involved in the production of *in vitro* embryos, embryo transfer or embryo-related technologies for breed improvement and conservation. Moreover, the OPU procedure does not interfere with the normal reproduction cycles of the donor; does not cause any detrimental effects on the donor cow's fertility. Besides, OPU technology has proved to be a reliable, repeatable and efficient technique for obtaining developmentally competent oocytes from live animal's viz. cattle (Pieterse *et al.*, 1988), horses, sheep, goats and buffaloes. In addition, oocytes could be recovered from normally cycling cows or hormonally pre-treated cows, clinically infertile or problem cows (Looney *et al.*, 1994 and Mishra, 2003), and buffaloes (Manik, 2003), pregnant cows, calves and prepubertal cows for *in vitro* embryo production.

After the initial development of the OPU technique, many studies were undertaken to investigate incremental improvements both in the technical and biological aspects of the technology. Technical aspects that were investigated included probe type, probe frequency, needle type, needle geometry, vacuum pump and pressure. Biological aspects investigated include donor animal herself, stage of the oestrous cycle, ovary and follicle size, OPU schedule (session/frequency), hormonal pre-stimulation, the experience of the operator. The main development in the OPU research is the use of hormones for super-stimulation prior to OPU, which yields greater advantages in terms of more follicles to aspiration, higher oocyte recovery rate and more embryos, and less work as compared to non-super stimulated OPU. Thus, the progress of research in this field lead to better understanding of optimal OPU schemes and *in vitro* embryo production system.

The ban on cow slaughter for religious reasons in our country makes ovum pick up (OPU) from live cows, the only technique available for obtaining cattle oocytes on a large scale from indigenous and crossbred cattle of high genetic merit. However, in India, the OPU technology is still in the infancy stage and scattered reports/works are available from NDRI, Karnal, TANUVAS, Chennai, GBPUAT, Pant Nagar, PGIVAS, Akola, NDDB NIANP and recently, by a private sector Bovageneix (JK trust).

Equipment and Procedure

Assembled OPU unit showing ultrasound monitor, transvaginal probe, needle, vacuum pump and oocyte collection system and tube (Jeyakumar, 2004).

The requirement of USG-TVFA-OPU comprises of an ultrasound scanner with a transvaginal transducer (probe), needle guide and vacuum pump. Real-time B-mode scanners (ALOKA 500 V, PIE MEDICAL 100 S/200 VET, SONOVET/SONOACE 600 V MEDISON / KRETZTEKNIC) are generally used. Initially, for ultrasound scanning of cow ovaries, a sector probe (curvilinear/convex array transducer) and a human endovaginal sector transducer were used. With the advancement of technology, transvaginal sector probe, specially designed for large animal usage was developed and used. Fingertip probe was used for visualizing the ovary and collection of oocytes from 6 months old calves. Certain probe with aspiration line or puncture line appearing in the monitor helps in better guidance of OPU needle during aspiration. The probe frequencies in (MHz) used for ovarian scanning and for aspirating follicles were 5.0, 6.0, 6.5 and 7.5. Generally 50 to 55cm length single lumen needle with different gauge viz., 17G, 18G, 19G, 20G and 21G were used. For transvaginal aspiration of ovarian follicular contents, most of the researchers used electrically regulated vacuum pump (K-MAR-5000/V-MAR-5000-Cook), hand operated non electrical vacuum pump (Jeyakumar, 2004) for vacuum generation and follicles were aspirated at a vacuum level ranging between 40, 50 and 72 to 100 mmHg with a flow rate of 12 to 22ml/min.

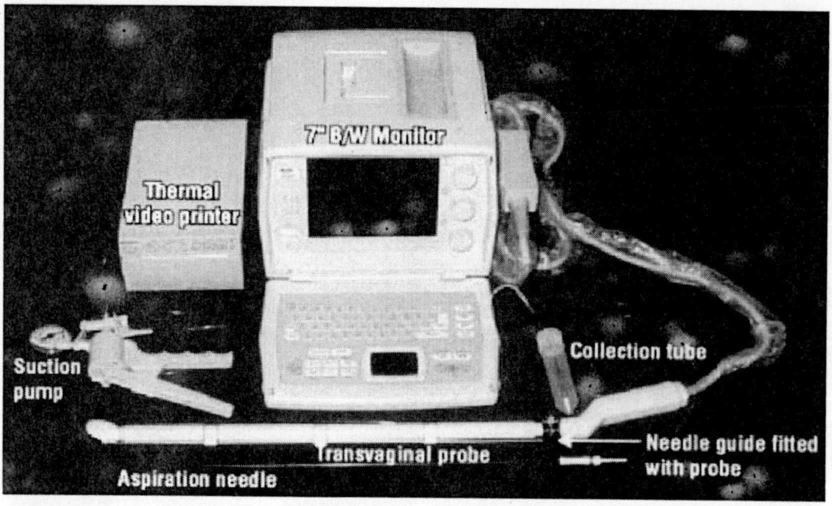

Assembled OPU unit showing ultrasound monitor, transvaginal probe, needle, vacuum pump and oocyte collection system and tube (Jeyakumar, 2004)

Efficiency of OPU

The efficiency of OPU can be measured through aspiration rate, oocyte recovery rate, and oocyte quality. Pieterse *et al.* (1988) suggested that the success rate of follicular aspiration could be measured, in part, by the number of immature oocytes collected from hormonally pre-treated or unstimulated animals in relation to the number of follicles present at the time of collection. The aspiration rate was calculated as the number of follicles aspirated expressed as a percentage of the total number of follicles counted for each cow. The oocyte recovery rate was calculated as the number of oocytes recovered expressed as a percentage of the number of follicles aspirated for each cow. Researchers classified oocytes into various grades, based on cumulus cell investment surrounding the oocyte, homogeneity and transparency of the oocyte cytoplasm.

Transvaginal ultrasound guided follicular aspiration (TUGA)-OPU

Impact on donors

1. Effect of OPU on oestrous cycle, follicular dynamics and on pregnancy rate
2. Ovarian changes
3. Epidural anaesthesia and stress

Factors affecting aspiration rate, oocyte recovery rate, oocyte quality and embryo production

A. Technical factors
   1. Probe type and its frequency
   2. Needle geometry
   3. Vacuum pressure

B. Biological factors
   1. Donor animal (age, reproductive soundness, pregnancy)
   2. Stage of the oestrous cycle
   3. Ovary and follicle size
   4. Ovum pick up a schedule (frequency/session interval)
   5. Hormonal pre-stimulation
   6. Operator's experience

Applications of OPU technology

1. OPU technology is low-invasive and well-tolerated by animals and adaptable to on-farm applications
2. OPU technology helps to selecting elite animals for embryo production
3. OPU yields a large quantity of oocytes from a single donor (as many as 1000 oocytes resulting in 300 embryos from a normal cow - Kruip *et al.*, 1994)
4. OPU/IVP has clear advantages over MOET and AI in terms of number of offspring that can be produced per cow per time span (on average for AI 1 calf per year, for MOET 20-25 calves per year, and for OPU/IVP 80-100 calves per year–van Wagtondonk-de Leeuw, 2006)

5. OPU technology is less dependent on the reproductive status of the donor cow
6. OPU technology does not require any exogenous hormones routinely, however, usage improves the efficiency of the programme
7. OPU has therapeutic value in infertile animals
8. Oocytes can be harvested from juvenile animals, heifers and from pregnant cows in the first three months of pregnancy
9. OPU/IVP offers a unique advantage as several bulls can be used for IVF on oocytes from one collection, rather than one bull as in MOET, thus maximizing genetic gain and minimizing inbreeding
10. OPU/IVP offers the possibility of doing IVF using sexed bovine sperm
11. OPU technology makes available, immature oocytes at places, where access to the slaughterhouse is limited
12. OPU technology can be employed as a research tool to study the physio-pathological events during follicular dynamics and oocyte development and intrafollicular environment under normal or experimental conditions
13. OPU technology helps in producing a large number of oocytes/embryos for conducting advanced research in the field of gamete cryopreservation, gene expression, cloning and transgenics, *etc.*
14. OPU technology offers unique opportunity towards conservation of farm and wild animal genetic resources i.e. to establish **Heritage Gene Bank** (storing maternal gametes/oocytes or embryos of threatened breeds) or **Oocyte Bank** programmes.
15. OPU/IVP may be considered as the only viable technological option, where there is a ban on the slaughter of cows (India) and for rapid genetic improvement in the cattle (dairy) industry.

Limitations of OPU

1. Cost of the equipment
2. High technical expertise
3. High degree of laboratory support for IVEP system
4. The long-term effect on oocyte donor and ethical regulations
5. Species and breed specific variations

OPU in Cattle

The donor cow is restrained in a suitable holding chute and administered an epidural block. A convex ultrasound 5 megahertz (MHz) sector transducer is fitted onto the distal end of a specially designed plastic handle and used to visualize the ovaries on the screen of the ultrasound monitor. The plastic handle (with a latex protective covering) is inserted into the vaginal canal, and then the ovary is grasped per rectum and placed against the transducer in the vagina. Follicles are identified as black (hypoechoic) circular shapes on the monitor screen. An 18-gauge, 55 or 60 cm-long needle is inserted through the needle guide in the plastic handle. This needle is connected to a suction pump by means of polyethylene tubing that passes through an embryo filter or into a 50 ml conical-shaped test tube for collection of the follicular fluid containing the oocytes. The basic solution used for this procedure is PBS, with 10 per cent bovine serum, antibiotics and heparin added. Using this aspiration method, oocytes are recovered from 60 to 70 per cent of the medium to large-

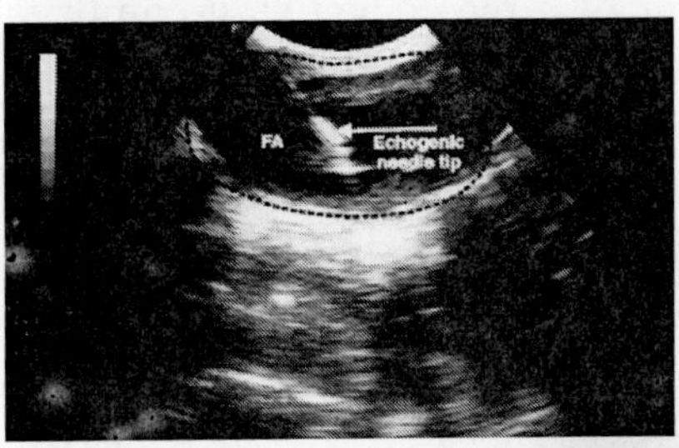

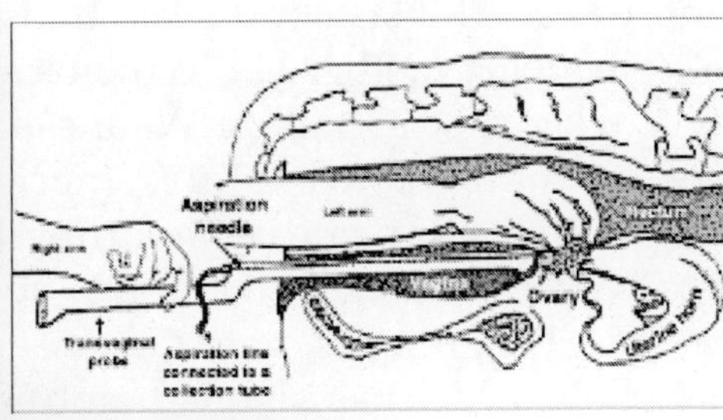

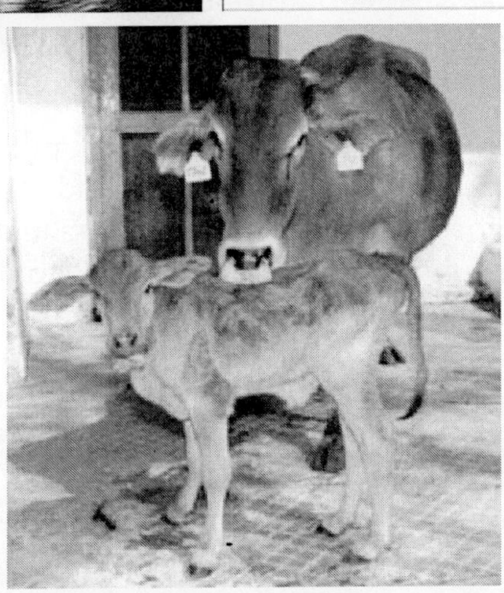

OPU-IVF, Calf "Holi" with surrogate mother

size follicles punctured, with an average of three to ten oocytes per non-stimulated donor female. A significant training period is required in order to become proficient in using this procedure in cattle. Aspirations are usually performed once a week but have been performed twice a week for up to three months in cows with no overt effects reported in the donor females. Manik *et al.* (2003) demonstrated the use of OPU as a means of obtaining developmentally competent oocytes from Karan Fries breed of cattle for obtaining cattle oocytes in India, where cow slaughter is not allowed for religious reasons. Jeyakumar (2004) concluded that increasing the frequency of aspiration (twice a week) was better than once a week group. Further, FSH pre-treatment of donors prior to OPU enhanced the overall OPU efficiency and *in vitro* embryo production rate in Jersey crossbred cows. India's first Ovum pick up – IVF cattle calf **'Holi'** born at ICAR-National Dairy Research Institute, Karnal. In OPU technology, oocytes were collected from the ovaries of a live Sahiwal cow using an ultrasound-guided needle. The oocytes were matured, fertilized and kept in an incubator for 7 days until development to a transferrable stage of embryo called 'blastocyst'. The transfer of a blastocyst stage embryo to a surrogate mother led to the birth of a female calf with a normal birth weight of 23 kg, on Wednesday, 7th March, 2012. The female calf is named as 'Holi' (accessed on 12.1.2017: http://www.ndri.res.in/ndri/documents/d37b12fe-3ecd-4b36-9a25-2efc2b67d018.pdf). Brazil is at the top of the list for embryos produced by OPU/IVP, besides other factors, there is a *Bos indicus* breed named as Nellore, which has a larger number of ovarian follicles with averages ranging from 18 to 25 recovered oocytes per OPU session without the use of exogenous hormones or synchronization protocols.

Through IVEP technology and well-planned crossbreeding programs, such as sexed semen and IVEP and transfer (SIFET) that integrate the use of indigenous cows as donors and surrogates while using semen from appropriate (more productive and reasonably adapted) dairy breeds, such as Jerseys, F1 heifers suited to the smallholder farmers conditions can be produced (accessed on 10.11.2017: https://www.ilri.org/ilrinews/index.php/archives/tag/sexed-semen-*in-vitro*-fertilization-and-embryo-transfer-project). Currently, OPU has been considered a promising technology and it has distinct advantages for rapid multiplication of germplasm for genetic improvement, breed conservation and provide basis for more advanced technologies, such as cloning and transgenics.

OPU in Buffalo

OPU-IVEP represents one of the latest assisted reproductive technologies used for faster multiplication of superior germplasm in buffalo. In buffaloes, considering the limited success on the application of MOET technology and IVEP using abattoir-derived ovaries the technique of ovum pick-up OPU-IVEP-ET seems to be a more efficient technology. The technique was first used in buffaloes by Boni *et al.* (1994) and birth of the first buffalo calf using OPU-IVEP was reported by Galli *et al.* (1998) and in subsequent years, more births were reported from different parts of the world (Infascelli, 2003 and Huang Y, 2005). The successful use of OPU for harvesting oocytes was reported in the swamp buffaloes, the Italian Mediterranean buffalo (Boni *et al.*, 1996) and the Murrah buffalo. **"Saubhagya"** is the first buffalo calf born through OPU-IVEP in India by Dr Shiv Prasad and his co-workers of Department of Veterinary Gynaecology and Obstetrics, College of Veterinary and Animal Sciences, G.B. Pant University of Agriculture and Technology, Pantnagar, India (Shiv Prasad *et al.*, 2013).

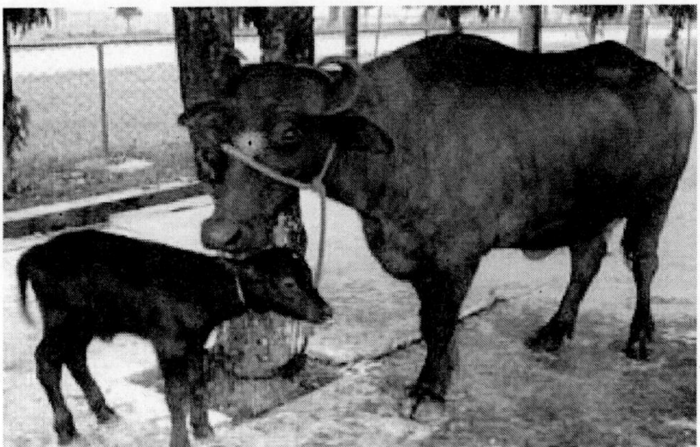

First OPU-IVF buffalo calf Saubhagya born at GBPUAT
(*Source:* Shiv Prasad *et al.*, 2013)

Liang *et al.* (2008), explored explore the use of sexed sperm and OPU-derived oocytes in an IVP system to produce sex-pre-selected bubaline embryos and suggested that OPU, sperm sexing technology, IVP, and embryo transfer, were used to produce sex-preselected buffalo calves. Further, this study provided proof of concept for further research and wider field application of these technologies in buffalo. It was demonstrated that twice-a-week OPU could be applied repeatedly, without any adverse effects on the follicular growth and oocyte recovery and that recovered oocytes could be used for *in vitro* embryo production in buffaloes (Manjunatha *et al.*, 2008) and in addition, the efficiency of OPU combined with IVP was higher during the peak breeding season than the low breeding season in buffaloes (Manjunatha *et al.*, 2009). Konrad *et al.*, (2017), evaluated the effect of the ovum pick-up (OPU) interval on follicular population, oocyte recovery, oocyte quality and *in vitro* embryo production and suggested to use a 14-days interval for oocyte collection in water buffalo.

OPU in Equines

Ovum Pick Up, Intracytoplasmatic Sperm Injection and Embryo Culture are techniques that can be successfully used in the equine industry to obtain embryos from mares that háve partially or totally lost their ability to produce offspring and in many cases represent the only option available. The same apply to stallions with low fertility *in vivo* or cases, when limited amount of frozen semen is available and it is not sufficient to perform artificial insemination. Embryos can also be produced outside the breeding season and frozen for later transfer, thus making this technique very flexible and versatile in a clinical setting. The pregnancy rate obtained in this retrospective study after non-surgical transfer of ICSI cryopreserved embryos is similar to those reported, when transferring fresh or cooled embryos produced by conventional embryo transfer and shows that the use of OPU-ICSI-IVC offers a real opportunity for breeding valuable stock in equine practice.

Ovum Pickup and Intra-Cytoplasmic Sperm Injection (ICSI) in horses: The technology of OPU-ICSI in equines indicated for, mares with reproductive problems (ovarian, oviductal and uterine pathologies) also related to ageing; mares with a history of recurrent abortions; mares in a competition that cannot carry a pregnancy; mares from which more foals or embryos are desirable; infertile stallions. There are currently two approaches to oocyte collection. One approach is the collection of mature oocytes. This is done by aspirating a large dominant follicle right before it ovulates and typically only one follicle is aspirated per cycle. The other approach is the collection of immature oocytes. In this approach, all the follicles that are present on the ovary at the time of the procedure, can be aspirated regardless of size because the mare does not need to be cycling. This approach results in a much higher number of oocytes retrieved but they must be matured in the lab. Statistically, the immature oocyte collection results in more pregnancies per aspiration but each mare are different and results may vary. As with any new technology, there is still a lot of information to be gained but we have done enough aspirations that we are comfortable saying this is a legitimate technology for the commercial breeding industry (Gabe Young, 2015) accessed on 12 Nov., 2017 http://info.selectbreeders.com/blog/ovum-pickup-in-the-mare. In conclusion, Ovum Pick Up, Intracytoplasmatic Sperm Injection and Embryo Culture are techniques that can be successfully used in the equine industry to obtain embryos from mares that have partially or totally lost their ability to produce offspring and in many cases, represent the only option available. The same apply to stallions with low fertility *in vivo* or cases, when limited amount of frozen semen is available and it is not sufficient to perform artificial insemination. Embryos can also be produced outside the breeding season and frozen for later transfer, thus making this technique very flexible and versatile in a clinical setting. The pregnancy rate obtained in this retrospective study after non-surgical transfer of ICSI cryopreserved embryos is similar to those reported, when transferring fresh or cooled embryos produced by conventional embryo transfer and shows that the use of OPU-ICSI-IVC offers a real opportunity for breeding valuable stock in equine practice. Ovum Pickup and Intra-Cytoplasmic Sperm Injection (ICSI) in horses (Barbacini *et al.* Accessed https://www.researchgate.net/profile/Denis_Necchi/publication/284408870, 412.pdf).

OPU in Small Ruminants

Laparoscopic Ovum Pick-Up (LOPU): One of the best techniques for oocyte recovery from live goats and was first described by Snyder and Dukelow (1974). OPU is considered as an efficient method for the genetic improvement, conservation and propagation high genetic groups of sheep and goat. The LOPU can be performed repeatedly over a valuable female cycling donor, pre-pubertal goats, infertile donor and does with a poor response on MOET and is considered as less invasive/traumatic and advantageous than laparotomy-based approach. In the recent period, OPU by laparotomy has been gradually replaced by LOPU technique in small ruminants (Rahman, 2008).

Transvaginal Ultrasound Guided Aspiration Technique (TUGA): OPU unit fitted with a 5 MHz transvaginal transducer is employed for OPU. In comparison to laparoscopic oocyte collection, TUGA has been considered as to be an alternate and safe method for

OPU. The oocyte recovery rate was comparatively less in TUGA than LOPU. Besides, the efficiency of TUGA-derived oocytes for IVP is not well-studied like LOPU.

OPU in Swines

Endoscopic ovum pick up (OPU) in swine is a minimal invasive and reliable technique to aspirate oocytes from preovulatory follicles for studying intrafollicular development and oocyte maturation as well as for IVM/IVF-programs (Brüssow *et al.*, 1997) and suggested that aspiration vacuum pressure of 17 to 32 ml water/min was found to be optimal in swine both for oocyte recovery and COC quality. Erena IKOMA (2014) reported that grade A oocytes are effectively retrieved with 90 mmHg of aspiration vacuum pressure and that application of the OPU technique enables us repeatedly to obtain embryos from highly valuable live pigs.

OPU in other Species

OPU has also been used successfully in other animals, with modifications made primarily to account for anatomical differences among species. For example, OPU been used successfully in adult pigs, llamas and various other hoofstock, such as red deer, sika deer, the rare bongo antelope and the African eland. Therefore, this technique may be particularly useful for managers of gene banks that preserve both domestic and wild animal genetic resources (*Source: Cryoconservation of Animal Genetic Resources, FAO, 2012).*

Conclusions

OPU can be considered mature technology and there will be a significant application of this technology over the next years for rapid genetic dissemination and conservation. Future research may be directed towards better understanding of *in vitro* embryonic development, to improve the pregnancy rates and to reduce LOS, peri/post-natal calf mortality.

References

Arun, V. (2003). Ultrasound guided transvaginal follicular aspiration and *in vitro* maturation of oocytes in cows. M.V.Sc. thesis submitted to Tamil Nadu Veterinary and Animal Sciences University.

Barbacini S., Colleoni S., Necchi D., Duchi R., Lazzari G. and Galli C. Clinical Application of Ovum Pick Up, Intracytoplasmatic Sperm Injection and Embryo Culture in Equine Reproduction Select Breeders Services Italia, Via Argine 39, 26046 San Daniele Po (CR), Italy. (Accessed on-line on 12.11.2017 https://www.researchgate.net/profile/Denis_Necchi/publication/284408870, 412.pdf).

Boni R., Di Palo R., Barbieri V., Zicarelli L. (1994). Ovum pick-up in deep anestrus buffaloes. Proc IV World Buffalo Congress; 3: 480-482.

Brackett, B.G., D. Bousquet, M.L. Boice, W.J. Donawick, J.F. Evans and M.A. Dressel. (1982). Normal development following *in vitro* fertilization in the cow, Biol Reprod 27, pp. 147–158.

Brüssow KP[1], Torner H, Rátky J, Hunter MG, Nürnberg G. (1997). Ovum pick up in swine: the influence of aspiration vacuum pressure on oocyte recovery from pre-ovulatory follicles. Acta Vet Hung. 45(2): 189-96.

Callesen, H., T. Greve and F. Christensen, (1987). Ultrasonically guided aspiration of bovine follicular oocytes, Theriogenology 27 p. 217 (Abstract).

Dellenbach, P., I. Nisand, L. Moreau, B. Feger, C. Plumere and P. Gerlinger (1984). Transvaginal sonographically controlled ovarian follicle puncture for egg retrieval, Lancet, p. 1467.

Erena Ikoma, Chie Suzuki, Yasuhiro Ishihara, Kikuo Komura, Tsutomu Ookoda and Hiroyuki Maruno (2014). Transvaginal Ultrasound-Guided Ovum Pick Up (OPU) in Berkshire Breed during Natural Estrous Cycle. Nihon Yoton Gakkaishi, 51(2): 45-53.

Gabe Young, (2015). Ovum pick-up in the mare. Accessed on 12 Nov., 2017 http://info.selectbreeders.com/blog/ovum-pickup-in-the-mare.

Galli C, Duchi R, Crotti G, Lazzari G. (1998). Embryo production by ovum pick up in water buffalo. Theriogenology; 49: 400.

Gleichert, N., J. Friberg, N. Fullan, R.V. Giglia, K. Mayden and T. Kesky (1983). Egg retrieval for *in vitro* fertilization by sonographically controlled vaginal culdocentesis, Lancet, pp. 508–509.

Hansen, P.J. and J.Block, (2004). Towards an embryo centric world: the current and potential use of embryo technologies in dairy production. *Reprod. Fertil. Dev.,* **16**: 1-14.

Huang Y, Zhang X, Gasparrini B, Presicce A. (2005). Oocyte recovery by ovum pick up and embryo production in Murrah and Nili-Ravi buffaloes (Bubalus bubalis) imported in China. Reprod Fertil Dev; 17: 273.

Infascelli F. (2003). First successful pregnancy from *in vitro* developed buffalo embryo. Bubalus bubalis; 9: 23-24.

J.Konradac, G.Cléricobc, M.J.Garridoac, G.Taminellib, M.Yuponia, R.Yuponia, G.Crudelia and M.Sansinenabc (2017). Ovum pick-up interval in buffalo (*Bubalus bubalis*) managed under wetland conditions in Argentina: Effect on follicular population, oocyte recovery, and *in vitro* embryo development. Anim. Reprod. Sci., Volume 183, August 2017, Pages 39-45.

Jeyakumar, S. (2004). Ultrasound guided transvaginal follicular aspiration and *in vitro* embryo production in cows. Ph.D., thesis submitted to Tamil Nadu Veterinary and Animal Sciences University.

Kruip, Th.A.M., R. Boni, Y.A. Wruth, M.W.M. Roelofsen and Pieterse, (1994). Potential use of ovum pick-up for embryo production and breeding in cattle. *Theriogenology,* 42: 657-684.

Liang X.W., Lu Y.Q., Chen M.T., Zhang X.F., Lu S.S., Zhang M., Pang C.Y., Huang F.X., Lu K.H. (2008). *In vitro* embryo production in buffalo (Bubalus bubalis) using sexed sperm and oocytes from ovum pick up. Theriogenology. 15; 69 (7): 822-6. doi: 10.1016/ j.theriogenology. 2007.11.021. Epub 2008 Mar 11.

Looney, C.R., B.R. Lindsey, C.L. Gonseth and D.L. Johnson, (1994). Commercial aspects of oocyte retrieval and *in vitro* fertilization for embryo production in problem cows. *Theriogenology,* 41: 67-72.

Manik R.S., Singla S.K., Palta P. (2003). Collection of oocytes through transvaginal ultrasound-guided aspiration of follicles in an Indian breed of cattle. Anim Reprod Sci. 15; 76(3-4): 155-61.

Manik, R.S. (2003). Transrectal and transvaginal ultrasonography with special focus on ovum pick-up in bovines, in manual on Ovum pick-up technology for *in vitro* production of embryos from elite farm animals, Division of physiology and climatology, IVRI, pp. 25-29.

Manjunatha B.M., Ravindra J.P., Gupta P.S., Devaraj M., Nandi S. (2008). Oocyte recovery by ovum pick up and embryo production in river buffaloes (Bubalus bubalis). Reprod Domest Anim. 43(4):477-80. doi: 10.1111/j.1439-0531.2007.00939.x. Epub 2008 Feb 17.

Manjunatha B.M., Ravindra J.P., Gupta P.S., Devaraj M., Nandi S. (2009). Effect of breeding season on *in vivo* oocyte recovery and embryo production in non-descriptive Indian river buffaloes (Bubalus bubalis). Reprod Domest Anim. 111(2-4):376-83. doi: 10.1016/ j.anireprosci.2008.03.003. Epub 20 Mar., 2008.

Meiyu Qi1, Yuchang Yao, Hong Ma, Jiabo Wang, Xiaochuan Zhao, Li Liu, Xiaodong Tang, Lili Zhang, Shengli Zhang and Fang Sun (2013). Transvaginal Ultrasound-guided Ovum Pick-up (OPU) in Cattle. J Biomim Biomater Tissue Eng 2013, 18:2, http://dx.doi.org/10.4172/1662-100X.1000118

Mishra, A.K. (2003). Ovum pick-up from infertile farm animals, in manual on Ovum pick-up technology for *in vitro* production of embryos from elite farm animals, Division of physiology and climatology, IVRI, pp. 34-40.

Pieterse, M.C., K.A. Kappen, Th. A.M. Kruip and M.A.M. Taverne, (1988). Aspiration of bovine oocytes during transvaginal ultrasound scanning of the ovaries. *Theriogenology,* 30: 715-762.

Rahman, A.N.M.A., R.B. Abdullah and W.E. Wan-Khadijah, (2008). Recovery and Grading of Goat Oocytes with Special Reference to Laparoscopic Ovum Pick-up Technique: A Review. *Biotechnology,* 7: 612-622.

Shiv Prasad, Beerendra Singh, Sumit Singhal, FA Khan, JK Prasad, HP Gupta, (2013). Production of the first viable ovum pick-up and *in vitro* embryo produced (OPU-IVEP) buffalo calf in India. Asian Pacific Journal of Reproduction 2013; 2(2): 163-165, doi: 10.1016/S2305-0500(13)60139-6

van Wagtondonk-de Leeuw, (2006). Ovum Pick Up and *in vitro* Production in the bovine after use in several generations: A 2005 status, Theriogenology, Volume 65(5): 914-925.

❑❑❑

Chapter 12

ETT: A Practical Approach for Conservation of Indigenous Germplasm

D. Saravanan

Artificial insemination (AI) has been in practice for breeding cows for nearly five decades. But, through AI, only 5-10 calves can be produced from an elite cow in a period of 10 to 15 years. However, from a genetically superior cow, nearly 20-30 calves can be produced in one year through Embryo Transfer Technology (ETT). ETT offers better utilization of superior germplasm of the female donor cow to produce a maximum number of high yielding offspring in a short period of time. A donor cow is made to superovulate and is bred through the semen of a superior bull, and 7-days old embryos from a donor cow are collected by non-surgical technique. These embryos will be transferred to the recipient cows, which will develop the fetus during the remainder of the pregnancy. Excess embryos can be stored in the frozen state for future use.

The benefits of embryo transfer technology are: (1) A high yielding cow may produce 8-10 calves in its lifetime by artificial insemination, whereas, 20-30 calves can be produced through embryo transfer technology in one year. (2) Elite cows have a significant role in enhancing the genetic potential of the herd through embryo transfer technology, like the genetic improvement of the herd by bulls through artificial insemination. (3) Embryo transfer technology reduces the transmission of infection from one herd to another. (4) Embryo sexing has the advantage in selecting the sex of the offspring before the transfer of embryos.

In India, there are 43 recognized breeds of cattle and 16 buffalo breeds. The population of the indigenous cattle has declined due to the cross-breeding programme, being uneconomical to maintain indigenous cattle breeds and mechanization of agricultural activities. The main advantages of indigenous cattle are: (1) Disease resistance,

(2) Low maintenance cost, (3) Better survival in the native tract, and (4) Drought resistance. Hence, it is essential to conserve and propagate the indigenous cattle breeds.

At DLF, Hosur, embryo transfer technology is practised in Red Sindhi cattle for the conservation of this breed. Red Sindhi cattle breed is one of the milch breeds of India. However, in India, there are only less than 1000 head counts of Pure Red Sindhi cattle, which are maintained only in a few government farms like Chiplima-Odisha, Kalsi-Uttarakhand, District Livestock Farm-Hosur. According to the National Bureau of Animal Genetic Resources, Karnal, Red Sindhi cattle breed is categorized under threatened breeds of cattle. Due to the cross-breeding programme, purity of this breed has declined over the years. As Red Sindhi breed is considered a milch breed of India, we do not have enough population of this breed, and we are in an urgent situation to multiply this milch breed through an Embryo Transfer technology in a short period of time. The Red Sindhi breed is heat resistant, tick resistant, and disease resistant, and can withstand extreme nutritional stress. As nearly 62% of our farmers are landless and depend on grazing their cows, Indian milch breed like Red Sindhi is ideal for our farmers. The cost of maintenance is very less, when compared to exotic cattle breeds, and the cows produce at least 2000 to 2500 kgs of milk in a lactation. The infertility problem is very less in this breed, when compared to the exotic breeds. The fat and SNF of milk of Red Sindhi cow is higher than exotic cattle breeds.

At District Livestock Farm (DLF), Hosur and in the farmers' cows of 12 districts of Tamil Nadu, the embryo transfer programme has been implemented. In the programme, so far, 251 cows have been superovulated and 1247 transferrable embryos have been produced, transferred to 1038 recipients and 333 pregnancies have been confirmed. Fifty three cows became pregnant through the transfer of frozen embryos and so far, forty calves have been born. **Altogether 251 calves have been produced and 41 cows are yet to deliver. Still, the field programme is going on, and by the end of this year, around 290 calves will be produced.**

Red Sindhi cows from DLF, Hosur of above 2500 kgs in lactation were selected as donor cows for embryo production. Cross-bred and poor milk yielding cows (otherwise healthy) were selected as recipient cows to carry the embryos of the donor cows till parturition. These donor and recipient cows were screened for infectious diseases like

Tuberculosis, Brucellosis and Johne's diseases and were given additional concentrate feed for one month to keep the cows in positive energy balance.

1. Selection of donors

A cow with high genetic potential and good cow index having completed at least one lactation should be selected as a donor. Milk recording of morning and evening on the first of every month for at least minimum of first ten months after calving is mandatory to assess the lactation yield of the donor cow. The donor should have completed minimum 60 days post-partum, so as to allow the complete involution of the uterus and attain normal reproductive hormonal profiles.

Negotiability of the cervix must be ensured and if required, cervical dilator may be used. The kinked cervix must be avoided. AI gun shall be used to ensure the patency of the cervix.

Since the recruitment of follicles following gonadotrophin stimulation declines with the age of the animal, the donors selected should be young, as the older animals (> 10 years) yield less usable embryos. Donor cows must be in second to the fourth lactation, and not beyond 7 years of age.

Records on reproductive cyclicity of the animals have to be checked for its regularity before selecting them for the programme. Non-cyclic animals can also be used as donors by using various progestagens. Infertile, anestrous, obstetrical or gynaecological problems must be avoided. Very small ovaries, ovaries with cyst, very long pendulous uterus must be avoided. Cows, which have calved more than one year, shall not be selected, as these cows may have an infertility problem. Health status of the donor has a direct correlation to the production of quality embryos. A very obese or very emaciated cow must be avoided. The animal to be selected as a donor should be free from major diseases viz., TB, JD, Brucellosis, Trichomoniasis, Campylobacteriosis, IBR and the donors are to be regularly tested for these diseases.

The donors should be in a positive energy balance. The donors should be neither overfed nor underfed, as both the cases yield poor superovulatory response. The donors in the field may be given additional concentrate feed of 3 kgs per day and mineral mixtures for one month.

2. Selection of recipients

Selecting a cow or a heifer as the recipient has its own advantages and disadvantages. There is less difficulty in calving in the case of cows, conversely, the heifers are easier to manage and have higher fertility rates. The choice of using the animal should be backed up by careful analysis of the factors mentioned.

Apart from these, the general criteria to be followed in selecting the recipients are:

- Be cycling regularly and should be in a positive plane of nutrition
- Have crossed 60 days of the postpartum period, but not more than 6 months, which is an indication of having infertility
- Have the ability to carry the pregnancy to full term
- Should not have any sort of reproductive anatomical abnormalities
- Better to have a thin uterus than a very thick and tortuous uterus, which will be very difficult to transfer the embryo without causing trauma to the endometrium
- Negotiability of the cervix must be ensured and if required, cervical dilator may be used
- Be free from abortifacients and diseases, as mentioned for the selection of donors
- Be docile and housed in close proximity for easier handling during the programme and effective oestrus detection.

3. Oestrus detection

Oestrus detection is both art and science. All the embryo transfer activities revolve around the onset of behavioural oestrus, therefore, the accuracy of oestrus detection holds the key for the successful embryo transfer.

The best and simple method to detect animals in oestrus would be to observe for the mucus discharge from the external genitalia while the cattle are resting or lying down. Alternatively, they can be observed for the two striking features viz., 'mounting other cows' and 'standing to be mounted'.

4. Superovulation

Meticulous care should be taken to see that the selected donor for the embryo transfer programme is utilized appropriately in such a way that maximum numbers of good quality oocytes are ovulated, they are fertilized and good quality embryos are recovered. This superovulation can be brought about by administering gonadotrophins at the proper time during the estrous cycle. The veterinarian and his team should follow superovulatory treatment protocol, based on the species, breed and type of the hormone to be used.

Care should be taken that the gonadotrophins used in the treatment schedule comply to the international safety standards. Gonadotrophins and other synchronization hormones are to be purchased from the reputed firms, the potency and batch number examined recorded and expiry is to be checked. Sterile procedures should be followed while injecting the hormones.

The re-constituted FSH should be preserved under refrigeration and the required quantity of hormone alone shall be taken in a syringe out of the refrigerator for injection. If there are two donor cows, a single vial shall be re-constituted first and the second vial after the completion of the first vial.

5. Selection of sire

Since half the genetic makeup of the progenies come from a male, it is extremely important to use genetically superior bulls. More care should be taken in selecting the sires as they will be mated with a large number of donors and any lacunae in this will prove costly. The sire selected should comply to the minimum standard protocol established for the breeding bulls (refer MSP for semen stations) in terms of the pedigree and disease testing.

6. Insemination

The very sterile procedure should be adopted while inseminating the animal by using the protective sanitary sheath over the AI gun. Due to more number of follicles present in the ovaries, care should be taken not to handle the ovaries either intentionally or accidentally during AI.

The time, when the donor is first observed in oestrus (after the superovulatory treatment) is the reference point for insemination. Since multiple follicles ovulate over a period of time and transport of sperm and ova are altered by superovulatory treatment, animals should be inseminated minimum two or three times at 12-hours interval between each insemination. The ideal time for insemination is 12 hours after standing the heat.

7. Recovery of embryos (Non-surgical method)

The non-surgical method of recovering embryos in cattle came into vogue from the late seventies. The protocol to be followed in the non-surgical method of recovering embryos in cattle and buffaloes are as follows:

- The recovery of embryos is generally carried out on Day 5½ to 6 and Day 7±1 (depending on the stage of the embryo to be recovered) from the onset of oestrus (Day 0) in the buffalo and cattle, respectively.
- Ovaries of the donor animal are palpated on the evening of the previous day of recovery and the number of corpora lutea in each ovary are ascertained so that logistical plans can be made.
- The donor cows shall be scanned for counting the number of CL on both the ovaries and also, any un-ovulated follicle.
- The donor cow shall be starved overnight to avoid frequent defecation during the flushing procedure
- On the day of recovery, the donor animal is brought to the embryo collection yard and secured in the flushing chute.
- The hindquarters especially the perennial area of the animal is thoroughly scrubbed and washed with iodine soap/mild soap to avoid any dung, mud, loose hairs and debris which may cause contamination during recovery of the embryos.
- Meanwhile, the complete assembly inclusive of consumables and instruments is arranged and kept ready in the tray.
- Lower epidural anaesthesia is given to the donor after back-racking the dung from the rectum. The dose of anaesthesia is decided in a manner that the animal loses its sensibility alone and does not become recumbent. A maximum of 2.5 ml of lignocaine 2% is sufficient.
- The onset of anaesthesia is characterized by flaccidity of the tail and the same is secured properly.

- Care to be taken by the operator that ballooning of the rectum does not take place, which causes difficulty in handling the organs.
- The vulvar lips are swiped with swabs dipped in 70% alcohol and allowed some time to dry, as the alcohol is extremely toxic to embryos.
- Better to avoid any disinfectants for cleaning the vulvar region, as these disinfectants and alcohol are toxic to embryos. Washing with clean water is sufficient.
- The catheter, preferably 18 F with six holes at the tip (appropriately chosen) is checked for the patency of the balloon and a sterile stylet is inserted into the lumen of the catheter and then rinse the catheter by flushing media.
- Care to be taken while passing the catheter into the uterus and fixed in the horn of uterus by causing no damage to the endometrium. The catheter should be taken until the anterior one-third of the uterus.
- For the inflation of the cuff, 5 to 6 ml of flushing medium can be used instead of air.
- Cervical dilators can be used prior to passing the catheter in case of difficulty in negotiating the cervix.
- The horns of the uterus are flushed with the flushing medium (D-PBS + 0.1% lyophilized BSA or 1% FCS maintained at 37°C) infused in an intermittent way and the embryos from the uterine horns are washed along with the fluid and are collected in the embryo filtering device.
- The filter shall not be dried or overfilled. A minimum of 30 ml of fluid shall be maintained in the filter always.
- The uterine horns can be gently massaged along with the fluid to dislodge the embryos attached to the endometrial folds.
- Excess of fluids being flushed into the uterine horn should be avoided. Overfilling of the uterine horn with fluid, without evidence of free return flow may cause endometrial or uterine rupture. Excessive uterine manipulation must be avoided.
- The uterine side with many CL on the ovary shall be flushed first, followed with the other side of the uterus.

- After the horn flushing, the cuff shall be deflated, brought near the internal os and again inflated with 2-3 ml of flushing medium keeping the cuff at the body of the uterus. Now, the flushing medium should be allowed to pass through both the horns and the medium should be drained out. Such body flushing shall be repeated three to four times. Finally, the flushing medium shall be left in the uterine horn keeping the catheter in the body of the uterus, and the outlet of the catheter is clamped.
- After the searching of the embryos, again the Y Junction tube is connected to the catheter, and the flushing medium in the uterus shall be drained out. Again, two body flushing shall be repeated.
- If the filter is blocked in between the flushing, a sterile 20 ml syringe (BD syringe without rubber plunger) can be used to remove the mucus and other debris blocking the filter, and the content is poured into a 90 mm Petri dish.
- The catheter should not be pulled out from the place of fixation before relieving the air or fluid from the balloon.
- The entire process of recovery must be done in sterile and hygienic conditions.
- Both the animal and the person, who does the recovery, should be comfortable and safely secured.
- After the recovery of embryos, the animal should be given an intra-uterine or intramuscular treatment of antibiotics and prostaglandin injection intramuscularly.

8. Isolation and handling of embryos

Contamination of air with disinfectants, odours, fly spray, chlorine or smoke is hazardous to the embryos. Excessive movement of personnel inside the laboratory must be restricted.

The embryo filter with 75 microns pore size is used to collect the embryos. The filtered content is transferred into the sterile 90 mm Petri dishes inside the laboratory and maintained under the laminar air flow unit. Dishes, which are not under examination, should be covered and protected from light.

The filter is washed in a manner so that the embryos and debris are dislodged from the sieve of the filter with flushing medium three to four times and the contents are taken in the searching dish having a grid at the bottom.

The filter with the lid is gently rotated clockwise and anti-clockwise for at least five times and the content is poured into the 90 mm Petri dish. The mucus in filter shall be aspirated using a sterile 20 ml plastic syringe without a rubber plunger (BD syringe is good). The nozzle of the syringe shall be moved in a circular fashion all over the filter to remove the debris and mucus.

Embryos should not be left in the original collection medium for longer than necessary since there may be substances present in the uterine flushing that can inhibit development. In addition, exposure to bright light, other than illumination required for microscopy, should be avoided in view of the evidence that daylight and ultra-violet light, in particular, may be harmful to embryos. A separate set of dishes and pipettes should be used to handle embryos from each donor to prevent contamination and inadvertent mixing of embryos. Careful labelling of dishes and pipettes will help to assure that this segregation is maintained.

The searching dish containing the uterine flushing is to be examined under the stereo zoom microscope under 10-20X magnification. Using the embryo picking device, the embryos are to be isolated and transferred to a dish containing holding medium (HM; D-PBS with 0.4% BSA or 10% FCS, which is filtered with 0.22 micron syringe filter) in a 35 mm Petri dish.

9. Washing of the embryos

Since only embryos with intact zona pellucida and free of adherent materials can be washed effectively, the embryos must be thoroughly examined over all their surfaces, and when necessary, any adherent mucus or other debris must be removed before washing. When defects of the zona pellucida are found or when adherent debris cannot be removed, these embryos should not be frozen, rather used fresh for transfer on the same farm. To confirm the intactness of the zona pellucida and freedom form adherent material, embryos must be observed over all surfaces at a magnification of 40-100 X. Essential requirements for proper washing of embryos:

- Only embryos from single donor washed together (confirm before washing)
- Ten or fewer embryos washed at one time (count before washing) **(Optional)**

- Minimum ten washes (allow sufficient time for thorough, gentle mixing in each wash) are required.
- Use a new sterile micropipette tip each time, when embryos are moved from one wash to the next
- Regulate (10 microlitres) volumes so that each wash is at least 100-fold dilution of previous wash

Washing procedures should always be completed before the procedures that invade the integrity of the zona pellucida like micro-manipulation, sexing and cryopreservation.

10. Evaluation and identification of the embryos

The grades/code in evaluating the embryos is strictly based on International Embryo Transfer Society (IETS) recommendations.

The embryos are to be evaluated under 40-100 X magnification of stereo zoom microscope. It should be recognized that the visual evaluation of embryos is a subjective evaluation of a biological system and is not an exact science. Furthermore, there are other factors, such as environmental conditions, recipient quality and technician capability that are important in obtaining pregnancies after transfer of embryos. There are different systems of grading the embryos. It is expected that qualified individuals, who grade the embryos will select the most appropriate code to match the condition of the embryo that they have observed. **Only Code 1 / Excellent /Good embryos should be utilized in international commerce.**

In general, the embryos are evaluated under four categories. The following points or criteria are to be looked into to arrive at correct evaluation: age (days post-oestrus), shape, cell number, compaction status, variability in cell size, colour of cytoplasm, areas of degeneration, numbers of excluded blastomeres (cells) size of peri-vitelline space, stage of embryonic development, and number of days the embryo is retarded from normal (e.g. a four-cell embryo recovered five days after oestrus would be two days retarded). After these are recorded, embryos are placed into one of the following categories:

- *Excellent or Good (Code: 1)*: Symmetrical and spherical embryo mass with individual blastomeres that are uniform in size, colour and density. At least 85% of the cellular material should be intact, viable embryonic mass. The judgement should be based on the percentage of embryonic cells, represented by the extruded material in the peri-vitelline space. The zona pellucida should be smooth and have no concave or flat surfaces that might cause the embryo to adhere to a Petri dish or a straw. The embryo should be consistent with its expected stage of development.

- *Fair (Code: 2)*: Moderate irregularities in the overall shape of the embryonic mass or size, colour and density of individual cells. At least 50% of the cellular mass should be an intact, viable embryonic mass.
- ***Poor (Code: 3):*** Major irregularities in the shape of the embryonic mass or in size, colour and density of individual cells. At least 25% of the cellular mass should be an intact, viable embryonic mass.
- ***Degenerating or Dead (Code 4):*** Degenerating embryos, unfertilized oocytes or 1-cell embryos: Non-viable.

It is often impossible to determine, if an embryo is a severely degenerated embryo or is unfertilized ovum. Even two or three-cell embryos may, in fact, be fragmented, unfertilized ova. Therefore, good experienced and skillful personnel are a prerequisite for the successful evaluation of embryos. As a rule of thumb, only good and excellent embryos are suitable for freezing and only fair, good, and excellent ones are suitable for transfer.

11. Loading of the straws

- The first step is to take a sterile 0.25 cc French mini straw, label it and rinse it twice with holding medium to remove any dust or toxic contaminants, taking care not to wet the cotton plug.
- An embryo picking device is used to load the embryos in a French mini straw. Embryos are loaded along with media in the manner so that on both the sides of the columns, there are air spaces/ columns, followed by the medium.

12. Identification of embryos

The identification of embryo is strictly based on IETS recommendations. All the bovine embryos are frozen in French mini (0.25 cc) straws. The labelling of the straws or the identification of the embryos is to be done as per the IETS guidelines. The information may be printed by hand or by machine on the straw, containing the embryo, on the extension of straw or plug (identification stick). It is recommended that two lines be used for labelling the straws.

13. Estrus synchronization

The most vulnerable principle of embryo transfer is that the stage of the reproductive cycle of the recipient must correspond to that of the donor or the physiological stage of the embryo. Perfect synchrony between recipient and donor is a must for good results. Ideally, the recipient should be in estrus on the same day as a donor. Asynchrony of one day may also be adjusted with the stage of the embryo.

There are many methods of synchronizing the reproductive cycles, of which widely adopted method is the administration of a luteolytic dose of prostaglandins or its analogue. All other methods of estrus synchronization, such as progestagens (CIDR, PRID) and Ovsynch treatment can be used. The choice is determined by cost and logistics.

14. Non-surgical transfer of the embryo

The evaluated good quality embryos are to be transferred into synchronized recipients to attain the end result of successful pregnancy and birth of a healthy calf. The most widely and commonly used procedure is the non-surgical method of transfer.

Lower epidural anaesthesia is recommended for routine non-surgical transfer. Manipulate the reproductive tract gently. The procedure for epidural anaesthesia is the same as for non-surgical embryo recovery. The embryo loaded ET gun, concealed in a sterile vaginal sanitary sheath, is passed upto external os of the cervix. The sheath is pierced and the tip of the ET gun is now passed at least up to the upper one-third of the uterine horn, ipsilateral to the corpus luteum. The embryo is transferred in a way that there is no damage to the endometrium.

15. Cryopreservation of embryos

There are a number of methods and machines that may be used for freezing and each describes specific procedures as well as provides sufficient descriptive literature for handling and use. Regardless of the method and procedure used, some points to be followed are :

- Embryos meant to be frozen should be thoroughly evaluated and only excellent/good embryos are to be frozen. For freezing, compact morula, early blastocyst and blastocyst stages are suitable. Morula and expanded blastocysts shall be avoided for freezing.
- Embryos should be washed in holding media in four-well Petri dish.
- All embryos should be examined under higher magnification (40-100X) for cracked zona and such embryos should not be frozen.
- Embryo straw (0.25cc) is to be rinsed, as mentioned under the loading of the straws.
- Embryos should be loaded in a straw and frozen quickly as soon as the grading is completed.
- If the embryos are to be frozen and transferred fresh, embryos must be frozen first, and then transfer fresh embryos to the recipient cows.

15.1 Conventional method of freezing

- Only excellent/good quality embryos are selected for cryopreservation after washing.
- The embryos are placed in the freezing medium (HM + cryoprotectant, such as 1.0-1.4 M glycerol/1.5M ethylene glycol, etc.), for the total period of 5-7 minutes at lab temperature (20-25°C) for glycerolisation.
- During this period, embryos are loaded into the embryo straws, as mentioned in the loading of embryos.
- The presence of embryo inside the straw is assured by examining the same under the microscope.
- While the loading the embryo into the straw, the programmable freezer is started and the freezing is carried out as per the freezing protocol mentioned by the manufacturer.
- Straw loaded with embryos are placed in the programmable freezer and are cooled down to -7°C and are held at this temperature for 5 minutes.

- The straw is seeded at -7°C by touching the supercooled forceps at the beginning of the first air column to initiate the ice crystal formation. Some of the freezing machines have auto seeding device.
- After seeding, the straw is held at the same temperature for 5 minutes.
- Then the temperature is brought down to -33°C to -35°C at the rate of 0.4°C per minute.
- After reaching the desired temperature, the straw is removed from the freezer and quickly plunged into liquid nitrogen.

15.2 Freezing with ethylene glycol (EG) method for direct transfer

This method has been used to circumvent to avoid thawing of frozen embryos in stepwise manner and microscopic re-evaluation of embryos under the field conditions:

- Only one embryo shall be transferred to the Ethylene Glycol medium at a time.
- While lifting the embryo from the holding medium, care should be taken to take a very minimal quantity of holding medium along with the embryo.
- After transferring the embryo into the EG, the medium around the embryo shall be rotated using micropipette for the thorough mixing of EG.
- Once the embryo is dropped in the EG, the timer must be set for seven minutes and shall be started.
- During this time, the straw should be labelled, and the details of embryo shall be recorded.
- After three minutes, the embryo shall be loaded in the mini straw with air column on both the sides of the embryo with EG medium.
- While sucking the embryo in the straw, it must be a quick suction so that the embryo comes at the beginning of the suction.
- After loading the embryo, the straw shall be looked under a microscope for the location of the embryo.
- If the embryo is at near the air space towards the opening of the straw, the straw shall be allowed to be in a vertical position for two minutes.

- Again, the location of the embryo shall be ascertained by looking under the microscope.
- If the location of the embryo is at the middle of the straw, then the straw shall be transferred to the freezer, which is kept at -6°C for two minutes.
- Later, the tip of the supercooled thumb forceps shall be touched on the straw with medium and embryo just below the air space for at least 10 seconds, which is called seeding.
- The time duration from the transfer of embryo into the EG medium to seeding shall be 7 to 10 minutes.
- It is very harmfulto the embryos to remain in the EG for more than 10 minutes.
- It is not advisable to transfer all the embryos into the EG medium at a time. By this method, some of the embryos would have spent a long time in the EG, which is not good for the embryos.
- So, while freezing, embryos must be transferred to EG only after the seeding of the previous embryo. So, only one embryo shall be processed for freezing, which will take 7 minutes.
- The embryo is packed in the straw in such a way that the central column contains 1.5 M EG with the embryo and the HM on either side. (a ratio of 1 part EG and 3 parts HM).
- The straws are either heat sealed or plugged with ET marking stick (plastic plug)
- Straws are transferred into programmable freezer and seeded at -7°C.
- Thereafter, the procedure is the same as that of the conventional freezing method.

16. Thawing of embryos

16.1. Conventional method of thawing

The first step in thawing is the removal of glycerol. A non-penetrating cryo-protectant like sucrose is generally used to maintain osmotic pressure during the removal of glycerol. The removal is done in three steps with decreasing concentrations of glycerol in HM:

i) A multi-well dish is used for thawing stepwise from first to the third step and the thawing media is filtered with 0.22m syringe filter.

ii) The straw containing the embryo is removed from the container after ascertaining its identity.

iii) The straw is placed in a water bath at 37°C for 30 seconds. Alternatively, air thawing can also be done to prevent zona damage.

iv) Wipe the straw and cut at one air space/column near the laboratory end.

v) The straw is held just above the well containing the solution of step I and the other end (factory plug) of the straw is cut near the air space/column, such that the embryo goes directly into the step I solution along with the freezing medium.

vi) The embryo is then transferred and allowed to remain there for about 5 minutes in each step.

vii) Finally, the embryo is placed in the HM for 15 minutes and re-evaluated for the quality to decide its suitability for transfer.

16.2 Direct thawing method

The straw containing embryo is removed from the container (as mentioned above), air thawed for seven seconds and thawed in a water bath at 30°C for 15 seconds. The columns are mixed and contents are transferred directly using the ET gun.

Abstract of ET

A total of 251 flushes were conducted in cows and a total of 1247 good quality embryos were collected (5.0 embryos/flush). Of these 1247 embryos, 1210 embryos were transferred to 1038 recipient cows, and 333 cows became pregnant (32% conception through both fresh and frozen embryo transfer). Of these, 231 cows delivered 251 calves (124 bull and 127 heifer calves) through embryo transfer technology. From the transfer of frozen embryos, 53 cows became pregnant, 37 cows delivered forty calves (14 bulls and 26 heifers).

For the conservation and propagation of Red Sindhi breed of cattle, which is an indigenous milch breed in the list of threatened Indian breeds, embryos of pure Red Sindhi cows and bulls were collected and transferred to cross-bred cows at District Livestock Farm, Hosur. Eighteen recipient cows delivered fourteen bull and four heifer calves.

The farmers are benefitted by getting incentives according to the number of embryos collected from their donor cows. The owners of donor cows were given an incentive of ₹ 5000 minimum for the first five embryos or a flush, and ₹ 1000 for every additional good quality embryo collected. A maximum of ₹ 26,000 was given an incentive to a farmer in Salem, whose cow gave 26 good quality embryos, out of 32 embryos collected. A total of ₹ 10.64 lakhs was given to 152 farmers, who gave their cows for embryo collection. Owners of the donor cows were given 90 kgs of concentrated feed free of cost. The donor cows also became pregnant after embryo recovery.

The owners of recipient cows were given 30 kgs of concentrated feed and an embryo from superior germplasm free of cost. If the cow becomes pregnant, an additional 150 kgs of concentrated feed was given to the owner of the recipient cow during the last trimester of pregnancy. If the cow delivers a bull calf, the animal husbandry department will purchase it from the farmer for ₹ 5000 within 15 days after its birth. If a heifer calf is born, the farmer can retain it. The animal husbandry department has purchased 98 bull calves from the farmers. The embryo transfer programme was funded by the National Project for Cattle and Buffalo Breeding through the Tamil Nadu Livestock Development Agency.

The highlights of the ET programme are

1. First field ET programme in India with more than 250 calves produced under field conditions.
2. Average of 5.0 embryo per flush
3. A maximum of 32 embryos from a cow in a single flush
4. Ten embryos from a donor cow were transferred to ten recipients in Theni district, and eight became pregnant and delivered eight calves in a single flush (four males and four females)
5. A maximum of 80% conception in fresh and 72% conception in frozen embryo transfer using farmers' cows
6. Forty calves were born through the transfer of frozen embryos
7. A total of 251 calves produced through ET (Male: 124, Female: 127).

Abstract of Embryo Transfer Programme as on October 10, 2017

No. of flushes	251
No. of transferable embryos	1247
Average No. of embryos/flush	5.0
No. of embryos transferred	1210
No. of embryos under storage	2
No. of embryos damaged	35
No. of recipients	1038
No. of cows verified so far	1038
Yet to be verified for pregnancy	0
No. of pregnant cows	333
Percentage of conception (Fresh & Frozen)	**32**
No. of cows delivered	231
No. of cows aborted	59
No. of cows sold/ died	2
No. of cows yet to deliver	41
No. of twin calves	20
No. of calves born (including twins)	**251**
Male	**124**
Female	**127**

❑❑❑

Chapter 13

Optimising the Intake and Feeding Management with Special Reference to Indigenous Cattle

Bandla Srinivas and Ajay Singh

Optimization is a process of finding an alternative with the most cost-effective or highest achievable performance under the given constraints. Optimum of any trait is a point, where marginal performance is higher and efficient in terms of resource utilization. This is contrary to either maximization or minimization, where consideration to resources is very little or nil. Optimization is restricted by the lack of full information. Feed intake, as one of the trait in the breeding program, optimization can possible only when genetic variability was higher in a population but not in a population under Hardy-Weinberg equilibrium. The objective of the present chapter is to optimize the feed intake and, secondly its management in indigenous cattle, where seldom systematic selection and breeding programs were executed (sparingly a little extent in limited breeds e.g. Sahiwal, Tharparkar).

Optimization of trait

Animals are described either in terms of appearance or performance or some combination of both. Traits of the animals are observable or measurable characteristic. If the traits are desirable, they need maximization, if not, minimization. In a biological system, minimization or maximization is followed to attain their potential suppression or expression, respectively. When the biological concept is amalgamated with sustainable development concept, economic prospects of either minimization of disadvantage trait and maximization of the advantageous trait would arise and weighed against resource input or output in proportion to input. Doctrines of economics emphasize that each incremental increase or decrease in a trait, the peak inflexion or deflection of incremented advantage or decremented disadvantage in relation to change in resources is considered to be more optimum. It is said to be optimum because each incremental increase or decrease will translate into a higher proportion of returns and point below which either the trait is not potentially exploited or above which the trait is exploited with disproportionate returns for the resources used.

Milk production is a good example to explain the influence of marker-assisted genetic selection that leads to maximization of herd average lactation yield to 10,000+ (Olsen *et al.*, 2002) in pure/graded Holstein Friesian cow. This genetic exploitation was criticized for compromising the fertility in *Bos taurus*. Such interpretations though appear simple but not free of any ambiguous assumptions. In the interpretation of cause and relation theories with the lesser assumption or free from assumptions are more preferred. The theory of theories 'Occam's razor' is often stated as an injunction not to make more assumptions than absolutely needed. This theory has a pleasing economy of its own: 'it is futile to do with more, what can be done with fewer'. In trait evolution, kind of argument has been used on both sides of the creationism versus evolution debate. Whether drawing 'the simplest explanation' under such complexity with minimum assumptions can be possible? If possible, is it 'usually the correct one'?

Optimization of trait versus Occham's razor

Genotyping and genomic selection have already enabled more accurate selection with a dramatically reduced generation interval compared with conventional selection systems based on daughter performance (Hayes *et al.*, 2009; VanRaden *et al.*, 2009). The level of complexity of most of the traits is great with the involvement of multiple genes and rapidly evolving knowledge on genomics, proteomics and metabalomics. Our present understanding in these areas and their interactions under molecular crowding at cellular levels are not adequate to undertake such comprehensive claim. Even a simple trait controlled by a single gene (e.g. Phenylketonuria in human–PAH gene, Hereditary Zinc Deficiency in cattle–SLC39A4 gene) appears to rapidly develop complexities beyond our current grasp because of a number of proteins, it may give rise. A viral proteome having 42 proteins encoded in their genome thought to interact each protein on average with 3 proteins. Thus, interactome may account about 126 interacting components. Out of which assume only 70% express and 30% are hidden (some are housekeeping and some are luxury genes). Even then, the interacting components are accounts to 88 proteins. Many hypotheses have been proposed to explain the complexity of gene expression by physiology, nutrition and management. These factors have been investigated at the animal, organ and cellular level at critical time points of the productive life of dairy cows (Walsh *et al.*, 2011). Often the concept of Occam's razor can also potentially mislead in genetics because one has to select the hypothesis with the fewest assumption among the competing hypothesis besides complex gene interactions. Although genetic improvement through cross-breeding increased lactation yield, dairy herds also posed difficulty in cows getting back calf at optimum intervals. This has lead to the presumption that inverse response in the fertility of dairy cow is a consequence of high milk production. According to Walsh *et al.* (2011), physiology, nutrition, management and immunology hypothesis are also cannot be overruled. Farm data indicated that the calving interval was only 20 to 32 days more than the average 407 d with lactation yield of 4000 to 6000 litres with every 2000 litres increase. Average calving index is also 420 to 438 d, when the herd average lactation yield ranged from < 6000 to 9000+ litres (Smith, 2010).

The Occam's razor also states that the simplest theory is best possible until simplicity can be traded for greater explanatory power. The observations of Smith (2010) are obviously trade-off the simplest theory that the increased milk yield affected the fertility. Generally, traits considered indicative of fertility has low heritability and metabolism of the animals is regulated less by gene and more by the metabolites (ter Kuile and Westerhoff, 2001). Therefore, metabolic changes or stress from the high milk production can be a credible reason with greater explanatory power to overrule simple presumption between milk production and reproduction. Hence, optimization of breeding programmes should take into consideration traits, their expression and metabolic implications with unavoidable construction of a biochemical network that links mRNA, proteins and metabolites (Brazhnik *et al.*, 2002). In general, the aim of the science is to seek the simplest explanation of complex fact may not possible in genetic improvement of animals but at the same time too many assumptions defeat the purpose of the solution. Henceforth, the complexity of genes controlling any trait needs to be explained without too many assumptions.

Feed intake

Feeding behaviour and the accumulation of energy stores are basic to the survival of all animals. Regulation of feed intake and energy balance in mammals involves similar regulatory and neural pathways (Kuenzel *et al.*, 1999). Regulation of feed intake has two key components: one that involves the short-term control of feeding and one that involves long-term regulation of energy balance by the central nervous system (Blevins *et al.*, 2002).

Dairy cows must consume large amounts of feed to provide necessary nutrients for their body to maintain growth, pregnancy, milk yield, etc. Therefore, dairy animals must have the capacity to consume dry matter without any physical or metabolic inhibitions. The utilization of the feed consumed by an animal involves a complex of biological processes and interactions with the environment. In addition, it is complicated by the fact that feed intake is highly correlated with body size and level of production. To overcome these complexities and to relate feed intake to production system efficiency, several measures of feed efficiency have been developed and used (Archer *et al.*, 1999). They can be grouped into gross efficiency, partial efficiency of growth, maintenance efficiency, cow/calf efficiency, etc. (Table 1). The concept of residual feed intake (RFI) presently preferred because it is an estimate of feed efficiency independent of the level of production (Alende *et al.*, 2016). Because RFI is by definition phenotypically independent of the production traits used to calculate expected feed intake, it allows comparison between individuals differing in level of production during the measurement period. This independence of RFI from production has led some authors to suggest that RFI may represent inherent variation in basic metabolic processes (Herd and Arthur, 2009).

Table 1: Definition of growth and feed efficiency traits

Trait name	Abbreviation	Definition
Live weight	LWt	Wt. at Specified age
Average Daily Gain	ADG	Wt. Gain per day
Relative growth rate	RGR	% change in the LWt/day
Kleiber ratio	KR	Wt. Gain / $kgW^{0.75}$
Feed intake	FI	Kg/d or kg/100 kg LWt.
Feed conversion ratio	FCR	FI/ADG
Partial efficiency of growth	PEG	Wt. Gain/(FI–FI for maintenance)
Residual feed intake (Based on feeding standards)	RFI_{fsf}	FI - Expected FI as per feeding standards
Residual feed intake by Regression	RFI_{reg}	FI - Expected FI as regression of average $LWt^{0.75}$ and ADG

B= Body, L= Live & Wt=Weight in kg: Ref: Arthur and Herd (2008)

A positive RFI means that the animals ME intake exceeds its predicted requirement for maintenance and growth indicating less efficient, whereas negative RFI indicates that animal either requires less energy than what is estimated or is eating less to produce the same weight gain (more efficient). It shows that efficient RFI heifers consumed less feed without any compromise in growth, body composition, or maternal traits measured (Lawrence *et al.*, 2011). Genetic variation in maintenance energy requirement per kilogram of metabolic BW was closely associated with genetic variation in RFI in young Hereford bulls (Herd and Bishop, 2000). In broad terms, there are likely to be at least 5 major processes, by which variation in efficiency can arise (Herd *et al.*, 2004). These are associated with variation in (1) feed intake, (2) feed digestion (and the associated energy costs), (3) metabolism (anabolism and catabolism associated with and including variation in body composition), (4) activity, and (5) thermoregulation. As feed intake increases, the amount of energy expended to digest the feed increases, in part because of an increase in the size of the digestive organs and increase in energy expended within the tissues themselves. Less RFI (greater efficiency) was associated with greater digestibility (Richardson and Herd, 2004). Compared to HF crosses, the 50% of sample size (N=50) in 3 experiments conducted on Deoni breed had negative RFI compared to 20% in HF crossbred calves/heifers (Table 2).

Table 2: Comparative RFI_{reg} in HF crossbred and pure deoni calves

Observations	Diet	HF cross calves		Deoni calves	
		RFI_{reg}	**MEI (Mcal)**	**RFI_{reg}**	**MEI (Mcal)**
1.	DCP 11% CPD 58% TDN 55%	**-103.78**	**7.30**	**-510.73**	**4.90**
2.		407.13	7.81	253.14	5.61
3.		343.80	6.55	440.04	5.85
4.		558.78	6.03	30.75	4.92
5.		363.09	5.90	85.25	4.43
6.	DCP 14.5% CPD 68% TDN 65%	127.77	8.82	**-231.86**	**5.25**
7.		492.57	8.46	**-194.20**	**5.69**
8.		0.06	9.30	**-225.86**	**5.00**
9.		0.34	8.27	142.30	4.58
10.		**-0.72**	**7.55**	**-67.21**	**4.27**

Metabolic body mass as selection criteria of breed

Sustainable livestock production is dependent on the utilization of the adaptive traits of indigenous livestock breeds. Many of the indigenous breeds of cattle are readily distinguishable from others due to their distinctive phenotypic features (Nahar *et al.*, 2016). The importance of selecting a breed or genotype, which is adapted to a specific environment in order to maximize efficiency and profitability has been stressed (Moyo *et al.*, 1996). Fertility and milk production potential of the dam are important factors affect weaning weight (Rutledge *et al.*, 1971). Calf weaning weight will contribute to the efficiency of the cow (Swanepoel and Hoogenboezem, 1994). Fertility, along with growth performance and lactation stress, offers a reliable measure of the degree to which an animal is adapted to a particular environment. Small body size is an adaptive attribute and considered that smaller cows tended to have lighter progeny due to reduced milk production. Reduced lactation performance has also been suggested as a contributing factor to improved fertility (Hetzel *et al.*, 1989). It is generally accepted that smaller cows are more fertile under extensive grazing conditions but larger cows produce more milk and wean heavier calves. Based on metabolically active tissue, the cow size of different indigenous and exotic breeds is shown in Table 3.

The main factors contributing to comparatively higher population variance in metabolic active tissue in indigenous breeds are lack of selection intensity, generation interval, genetic variation and accuracy of selection (Betz, 2007). Greater genetic variation in the metabolically active tissue in indigenous cattle is indeed, an opportunity to greater genetic change through selection. For example, selection for increased milk production in HF is a classic example. The amount of genetic diversity that remains in that population is minimal (<2% σ^2), leaving the breeder with limited opportunities for further genetic change in other quality traits. The juxtaposition of milk production with some of the quality traits may lead to sacrifice traits related to stress resilience, energy metabolism, fertility, etc., in breeds like HF (Shackelford, *et al.*, 1994).

Table 3: Population variance of breeds for metabolically active tissue.

Breed	Body weight (kg)		Metabolic BW ((kgW^{075})		Population Variance (%)
	Range	Mean	Range	Mean	
Exotic breeds					
Holstein	545-620	583	113-124	119	2
Angus	503-582	543	106-118	112	2
Hereford	490-590	540	104-120	112	3
Jersey	394-485	440	88-130	96	4
Indigenous breeds					
Deoni	325-485	400	77-103	89	16
Ongole	363-591	477	83-120	102	23
Gir	319-568	444	75-116	97	31
Sahiwal	301-544	423	72-113	93	33
Tharparker	293-544	419	71-113	93	36
Haryana	287-499	393	70-106	88	29
Red sindhi	317-454	386	75-98	87	13
Rathi	295-386	341	71-87	79	7
Malnad Gidda	80-120	110	27-36	34	13
Ponganur	90-130	100	29-38	32	26

Phenotypic limitation of the digestive system in indigenous cattle

The valuation of alternative scenarios in terms of phenotypes requires a number of assumptions. Additional phenotypes typically increase the accuracy of evaluation and resulting genetic gain. Phenotypic plasticity refers to the changes in animal behaviour, morphology and physiology due to its adaption to a unique environment. It is the ability of one genotype to produce more than one phenotype, when exposed to a different environment (Figure 1).

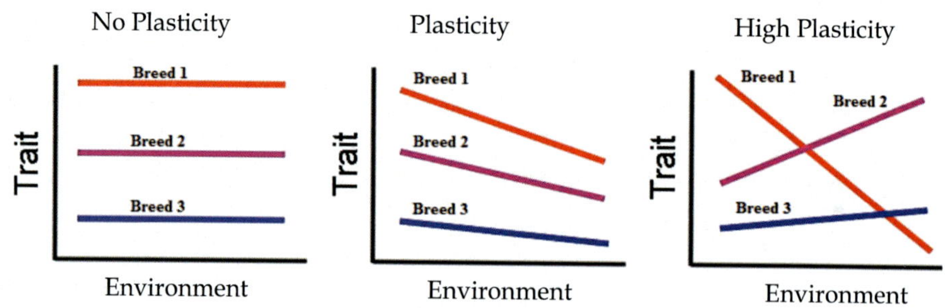

Figure 1: Phenotypic plasticity

Phenotypic plasticity in animals focused mainly on developmental effects of nutrition and temperature. One of the methods for its measurement is trait reaction norms. Plasticity of the digestive system of animals allows their response to changes in dietary nutrient composition, diet quality and energy requirement. Changes in the proportion of protein, carbohydrates and lipids in the diet are possible with the season and also during a major shift in physiological stages, for example, weaning, pregnancy, lactation, *etc*. Often, rumen environment fluctuations are controlled by the host cow and maintained a coordinal temperature and pH by self-regulated intake. Therefore, the plasticity of the digestive system is mainly concern to enzymatic digestion that is mediated by the digestive enzymes secreted by the animals. Animals, which can increase the activity of aminopeptidase-N, may able to acclimatize to high protein diets and show high plasticity (Cortés *et al.*, 2011). Poor quality diets, such as high fiber and low protein, have lower concentrations of nutrients. As a result, animals must process a greater total volume of poor-quality food to extract the same amount of energy as they would from a high-quality diet. Animal performance would be limited, when fail to respond to increase their food intake, enlarging digestive organs, and increasing the capacity of the digestive tract on a poor diet. Same shall be reverse with high protein diets. Poor quality diets may result in lower concentrations of nutrients in the lumen of the intestine and decrease in the activity of several digestive enzymes while, high protein diets may limit by enzyme secretion and comprise of dry matter intake to the level of saturation in protein intake.

A fundamental principle of nutrition and metabolism is that body weight change is associated with an imbalance between the energy content of diet consumed and energy expended by the body to maintain life and to perform physical work. Such an energy balance framework is a potentially powerful tool for investigating the regulation of body weight. Energy intake includes 3 major macronutrient groups; carbohydrate, protein, and fat with a smaller component coming from alcohol. Once ingested, the net absorption of the major macronutrient groups is variable and incomplete, with fecal losses accounting for 2–10 per cent of gross energy. Metabolizable energy expenditure for obligatory processes (digestion and processing of ingested food) has hierarchy of protein>carbohydrates>fat (Hall *et al.*, 2012). The ability of two distinctive genotypes; HF crosses and Deoni for normal diet and high density protein and energy supplement is presented in Figure 2.

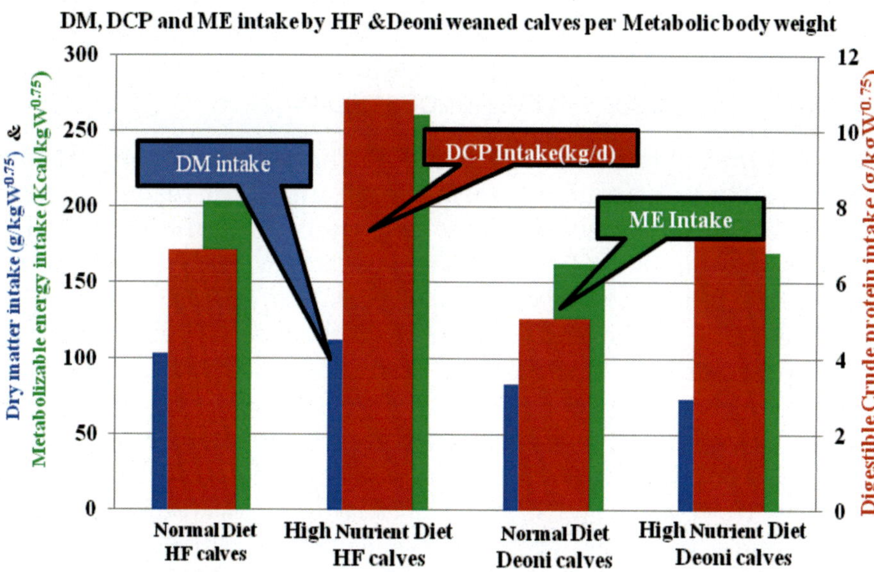

Figure 2: Phenotypic plasticity of the digestive system in indigenous and crossbred genotypes

In a study, conducted by Singh and Srinivas (2017) on 2 distinct genotypes; HF crossbred and pure Deoni calves, weaned HF crossbred calves consumed 40, 55 and 30 per cent more dry matter (DM), digestible crude protein (DCP) and metabolizable energy (ME) intake (I), when fed 10 per cent more CP and gross energy (GE) than normal diet having 16 per cent CP and 55 per cent TDN (1kg TDN = 3.8 Mcal). Weaned calves of pure Deoni breed consumed 9 and 34 per cent more DM and DCP over normal diet but, ME intake was reduced by 1 per cent. It is a classic example for poor plasticity of the digestive system of Deoni calves where high protein intake limited by the aminopeptidase-N in the digestive system. DMI of Deoni calves was curtailed to the level that is quantitatively equal DCP on a normal diet. Thus, genetically improved HF crosses were shown plasticity to nutrient quality and quantity $\geq$ 55 per cent. Those breeds (e.g. Deoni) which are deprived of genetic selection, were shown at the most 10 per cent plasticity. Although Deoni calves were consumed more protein, their diet was energetically imbalanced. Any imbalance between the intake and utilization of these macronutrients will lead to an alteration in body composition. The energy stored per unit body weight of carbohydrate, fat, and protein varies considerably, especially when accounting for the associated intracellular water (Hall *et al.*, 2012).

Metabolic limitations in indigenous cattle

RFI in different genotypes and genetic variance in animals may likely to vary because of variation in intake of feed, digestion, metabolism, physical activity and thermoregulation. Feeding management in the indigenous breed of cattle is hindered due to poor plasticity of the digestive system and portal drain viscera metabolism. The genetic and phenotypic relationship between insulin sensitivity, insulin-like growth factor and net feed intake was studied in relation to growth performance of calves (Moore *et al.*, 2005). Indigenous calves have low insulin activity compared to genetically improved HF crosses. Insulin sensitivity in young calves is associated with the change in muscle fiber areas with growth (Arthur and Herd, 2008). The maximum growth rate observed in weaned Deoni calves is 300 g/d (σ_x 36 g) compared to 500 g/d (σ_x 43 g) on mixed diets under Indian conditions, which indicate that the time delay between both the genotypes to achieve puberty is 30 to 60%. Weaned Deoni calves often experience problems in glucose homeostasis and shows post prandial hyperglycemia, which disappears with age and body weight gain. Indigenous breeds of lactating cow suffer low insulin concentration ($P < 0.01$) until 4th lactation. Plasma concentration of insulin in lactating

Deoni cows was 40.24 ±0.29 mg/dl (Srinivas *et al.*, 2010) in comparison to 65.68 mg/dl in ½HF×½Redi Sindhi (Chaiyabutr *et al.*, 2000). Plasma triglycerides were 58 % higher (P = 0.03) in Deoni than HF crossbred calves fed common diet. Simultaneously, the ratio between aspartate transaminase (AST) and alanine transaminase (ALT) was above 2:1 in Deoni calves compared to below 2:1 in HF crossbred calves. This is an indication of fatty liver, adipocytes breakdown and hindrances in energy metabolism in indigenous breed compared to HF crosses (Singh and Srinivas, 2017).

Epilogue

RFI is phenotypically independent of the production traits and represents inherent variation in basic metabolic processes individual animals. Number of indigenous cattle e.g. Deoni animals have negative RFI than crossbred calves/heifers (50% vs. 20%) thus, indicating animal either requires less energy than what is estimated or is eating less to produce the same weight gain (more efficient). However, the major setback of indigenous calves is very limited phenotypic plasticity of the digestive system and metabolism i.e., about 10% in comparison to ≥ 50% in genetically improved HF crosses. Phenotypic plasticity in digestion and metabolism in indigenous cattle need to be improved in the diverse population. Indigenous calves have low insulin activity compared to genetically improved HF crosses, thus, indicating a slow change in muscle fiber areas with growth. The higher ratio between aspartate transaminase (AST) and alanine transaminase (ALT) i.e., above 2:1 in Deoni calves compared to below 2:1 in HF crossbred calves is an indication of fatty liver, adipocytes breakdown and hindrances in energy metabolism. The maximum growth rate observed in weaned Deoni calves is 300 g/d (σ_x 36 g) compared to 500 g/d (σ_x 43 g) in HF crossbred calves on mixed diets, which indicate that the time delay in Deoni calves to achieve puberty is 30 to 60 per cent compared to HF crosses. Since feed expenditure accounts to 60 to 70% of variable costs on the farm, it is necessary to improve the plasticity of digestion and metabolism in indigenous cattle. Without which, small or large dairy farmers may show a lukewarm response to the idea of rearing indigenous cow breeds despite of launching subsidy-cum-training schemes encouraging to start *desi* cattle units.

References

Alende, M., P.A. Lancaster, M.L. Spangler, A.J. Pordomingo and J.G. Andrae, (2016). Residual feed intake in cattle: Physiological basis. A Review. *Revista Argentina de Producción Animal* 36(2): 49-56 (2016).

Archer, J.A., and S.A. Barwick, (1999). Economic analysis of net feed intake in industry breeding schemes. In: Association for the Advancement of Animal Breeding and Genetics, 13, 1999, Bunbury. Proceedings. Bunbury Association for the Advancement of Animal Breeding and Genetics, p. 337-340.

Arthur, P.F. and R.M. Herd, (2008). Residual feed intake in beef cattle. *Revista Brasileira de Zootecnia* 37: 269-279. http://www.scielo.br/pdf/rbz/v37nspe/a31v37nsp.pdf (DoA 21/06/2017).

Betz, G.M. (2007). Using the rate of change and the population structure of cattle to better target genetic progress. Symposium of Beef improvement federation. June 6 to 9th. 39th Annual meeting. Fort Collins, Colorado. Angus Production Inc. (Publ. and Copy right), 3201 Federick Ave, St. Joseph, MO 64506.

Brazhink P., A. de la Fuente and P. Mendes, (2002). Gene networks: how to put the function in genomics. *Trends Biotechnology*, 20: 467-72.

Chaiyabutr N., S. Preuksagorn, S. Komolvanich and S. Chanpongsang, (2000). Plasma levels of hormones and metabolites as affected by the forages type in two different types of crossbred Holstein cattle. *Asian Austalasian Journal of Animal Science* 13: 1359-1366.

Cortés P, A., M. Franco, P. Sabat, S.A. Quijano and R.F. Nespolo, (2011). Bioenergetics and intestinal phenotypic flexibility in the microbiotherid marsupial (Dromiciops gliroides) from the temperate forest in South America. *Comparative Biochemistry and Physiology. Part A, Molecular & Integrative Physiology*. 160(2): 117–124.

Hall, Kevin D., B. Heymsfield Steven, W. Kemintz Joseph, Kelin Samuel., A. Dale Scholle. and John R Speakman, (2012). Energy balance and its components: imnplications for body weight regulation. *Americal Journal of Clinical Nutrition* 95: 989-994.

Hayes, B.J., J. Pryce, A.J. Chamberlain, P.J. Bowman, and M.E. Goddard, (2010). Genetic architecture of complex traits and accuracy of genomic prediction: Coat colour, milk-fat percentage, and type in Holstein cattle as contrasting model traits. PLoS Genet. 6:e1001139 http://dx.doi.org/10.1371/journal.pgen.1001139.

Herd, R.M. and P.F. Arthur, (2009). Physiological basis for residual feed intake. *Journal of Animal Science*, 87: E64-E71.

Herd, R.M. and S.C. Bishop, (2000). Genetic variation in residual feed intake and its association with other production traits in British Hereford cattle. *Livestock Production Science,* 63(2): 111-119.

Hetzel, D.J. Mackinnon, M.J. Dixon, R. Entwistle, K.W. (1989). Fertility in a tropical beef herd divergently selected for pregnancy rate. *Animal Production* 49: 73-81.

Kuenzel, W.J., M.M. Beck, and R. Teruyama, (1999). Neural sites and pathways regulating food intake in birds: A comparative analysis to mammalian systems. *Journal of Experimental Biology,* 283: 348–364.

Lawrence, P., D.A. Kenny, B. Earley, D.H. Crews and M. McGee, M. (2011). Grass silage intake, rumen and blood variables, ultrasonic and body measurements, feeding behaviour, and activity in pregnant beef heifers differing in phenotypic residual feed intake. *Journal of Animal Science,* 89(10): 3248-3261.

Moore, K.L., D.J. Johnston and H-U Graser, (2005). Genetic and phenotypic relationships between insulin-like growth factorI (IGF-I) and net feed intake, fat and growth traits in Angus beef cattle. *Australian Journal of Agricultural Research* 56: 211-218.

Moyo S, F.J.C. Swanepoel and J.E.O. Rege, (1996). Evaluation of indigenous, exotic and crossbred cattle for beef production in a semi-arid environment: reproductive performance and cow productivity. *Proceedings Australian Society Animal Production* 21: 204-206.

Nahar, S., A.F.M.F. Islam, M.A. Hoque and A.K.F.H. Bhuiyan, (2016). Animal performance of indigenous Red Chittagong cattle in Bangladesh. *Acta Scientiarum. Animal Sciences Maringá* 38(2):177-182.

Richardson, E.C. and R.M. Herd, (2004). Biological basis for variation in residual feed intake in beef cattle. 2. Synthesis of results following divergent selection. *Animal Production Science.* 44(5): 431-440.

Rutledge, J.J., O.W. Robison, W.T. Ahlschwede and J.E. Legates, (1971). Milk yield and its influence on 205-day weight of beef calves. *Journal of Animal Science* 33: 563-567.

Shackelford, S.D., M. Koohmaraie, L.V. Cundiff, K.E. Gregory, G.A. Rohrer, and J.W. Savell, (1994). Heritabilities and phenotypic and genetic correlations for bovine postrigor calpastatin activity, intramuscular fat content, WarnerBratzler shear force, retail product yield, and growth rate. *Journal of Animal Science* 72: 857-863.

Singh, A. and B. Srinivas, (2017). Growth performance and immune status of weaned HF crossbred and Deoni calves with enhanced nutrition.

M.V.Sc., (Animal Nutrition) Dissertation. Southern Regional Station, ICAR-NDRI, Bangalore. Pp. 76-79.

Smith, R. (2010). Fertility and milk yield - can we manage both together? *International Dairy Topics*, 10: 23-25.

Srinivas, B., K.S. Prasad, A. Obireddy, I.J. Reddy, S. Selvaraju, and M.K. Rao, (2010). *Studies on nutritional, endocrinal and reproductive profiles in lactating Deoni cattle.* Institute Research Project under the program on Biotechnological augmentation of growth, lactation and reproduction in dairying, ICAR-NDRI, Bangalore. Pp. 1-22.

Swanepoel, F.J.C. and J.M. Hoogenboezem, (1994). Inter-relationship among cow size, lifetime cow fertility, milk production and pre-weaning calf growth in sub-tropically adapted beef cattle. *Proceedings Australian Society Animal Production*, 20: 78-80.

Tur Kuile B.H. and H.V. Westerhoff, (2001). Transcriptome meets metabolome: hierarchical and metabolic regulation of the glycolytic pathway. *FEBS Letter*, 500: 169-71.

VanRaden, P.M., C.P. Van Tassell, G.R. Wiggans, T.S. Sonstegard, R.D. Schnabel, J.F. Taylor, and F.S. Schenkel, (2009). Invited review: Reliability of genomic predictions for North American Holstein bulls. *Journal of Dairy Science*, 92: 16–24.

Walsh, S.W., E.J. Williams, and A, C. Evans, (2011). A review of the causes of poor fertility in high milk production dairy cows. *Animal Production Science*, 123: 127-138.

□□□

Chapter 14

Status and Prospects of Indigenous Cattle Farming in Southern India: Farmers Perspective

S. Subhash, K.P. Ramesha and M.C.A. Devi

Introduction

India has rich and diverse genetic resources of livestock population of about 512 million livestock and 729 million poultry birds (19th Livestock Census, 2012). Cattle rearing has been a traditional livelihood in India and is closely linked to the agricultural economy by providing the economical and nutritional security to our masses. Dairying has also been a livelihood for a large population of our country. About 70 million rural households are engaged in milk production, the majority being small and marginal farmers and landless. In our country, at present with about 191.90 million cattle has around 14 per cent of the world cattle population. Of this, 79 per cent i.e. 151 million are indigenous and only 21 per cent are exotic/crossbred animals. Most of the indigenous cattle (about 80 percent) are non-descript and only 20 per cent i.e. 43 indigenous breeds are recognized by ICAR-NBAGR, Karnal. Indigenous cattle are robust and resilient and are particularly suited to the climate and environment of their respective breeding tracts. Endowed with qualities of heat tolerance, resistance to diseases and the ability to thrive under extreme climatic stress and less than optimal nutrition, indigenous cattle plays a significant role in supporting the livelihood of smallholder dairy farmers through supply of milk, draught animal power, breeding purpose, and cow urine & manure, which has got medicinal value. In this regard, considering the importance of indigenous cattle, the Government of India has come out with 'Rashtriya Gokul Mission' aims to conserve and develop indigenous breeds in a focused and scientific manner during the 12th Plan period. It envisages that the potential to enhance the productivity of the indigenous breeds of India through professional farm management and superior nutrition is immense. For this, it is essential to promote conservation and development of indigenous breeds (Rashtriya Gokul Mission, 2014).

Indigenous cattle breed of Southern India

In Southern India, comprised of Andhra Pradesh (undivided), Karnataka, Kerala and Tamil Nadu possess around 10.80 per cent of total indigenous cattle population of our country. Out of 43 recognized indigenous cattle breeds, 13 are from southern India which includes Ongole, Punganur from Andhra Pradesh, Deoni, Hallikar, Amritmahal, Malnad Gidda, Krishna Valley and Khillar from Karnataka, Vechur from Kerala, Kangayam, Umblachery, Pulikulam and Bargur from Tamil Nadu.

S. No.	State	Total Indigenous Cattle Population	Per cent in Total Indigenous Cattle Population
1.	Andhra Pradesh	71,98,491	4.76
2.	Karnataka	66,03,967	4.36
3.	Tamil Nadu	24,59,548	1.62
4.	Kerala	77,045	0.05
	Total	**1,63,39,051**	**10.8**

Source: Breed Survey, 2012 MoA & FW, GoI

The latest livestock census clearly indicates that the total indigenous cattle population is declining to the tune of 8.94 per cent compared to the crossbred population, but still contributing 21 per cent of total milk production in our country with a marginal increase in milk production of our indigenous cattle. The major reasons attributed for its declining population is due to the indiscriminate crossing of native stocks and un-scientific cross-breeding policy adopted over the years. The other factors responsible for the loss of genetic diversity among livestock include loss of grazing land, globalization of the economy, catastrophes, conflicts, legal restrictions on marketing of livestock products, invasion of chemical inputs into agriculture, large scale mechanization of agriculture and transport, changing cropping patterns, degradation of forests, shrinking grazing and water resources, state-driven afforestation and Silvi-pasture programmes (Ramesha, 2013). However, despite its lower milk yield potential, our study indicates that, farmers at the field level perceive its importance beyond milk yield and attribute to its suitability to their resource-specific farming system, resistance to diseases, low maintaining cost and has higher economic value- which is being recognized in recent years, as the demand for antibiotic-free, clean and safe, organic milk is increasing among the health conscious consumers. Further, the growing concern among the farmers towards organic/natural farming, necessitates rearing of indigenous cattle for its quality dung and urine and hence, there is an increasing interest/tendency among the farmers towards rearing of indigenous cattle primarily for meeting their own home and farm requirements along with crossbred cattle for higher economic returns through sale of milk. In addition to this, due to the support under Rashtriya Gokul Mission, there is an increasing trend in the establishment of indigenous cattle based Gaushalas and individual farms as an enterprising activity by producing various products from cattle's dung and urine.

Present Status of indigenous cattle farming in Southern India

The field survey conducted on indigenous cattle farming system in Karnataka and Tamil Nadu states indicated that the majority of the farmers rear 2-3 indigenous cattle with an average milk yield of 2-4 litres/day along with HF crossbred cattle to support their livelihood. The indigenous cattle breeds were reared under semi-intensive management where in most of the cases the cattle were primarily allowed for grazing and then stallfed with available green grasses, paddy straw, ragi straw and other feedstuffs including concentrate feeds to the milch animals. The animals mostly were housed in a loose, semi-structured cattle sheds and maintained mostly in their home premises. The indigenous cattle from Karnataka, such as Deoni, Hallikar, Amritmahal were widely used for ploughing purpose as the majority of the respondents are smallland holders and found that it was very ideal for inter cultivation operations. For the breeding, majority of them resort to AI services and that leads to use of either Hallikar or Amritmahal semen as the availability of Hallikar semen is very limited. In the case of Malnad Gidda breed, unique indigenous cattle of Western Ghat, the farmers are rearing this indigenous dwarf breed with a low investment primarily for its quality dung to be used for their plantation crops and for its much-demanded ghee, which is sold for a premium price at the local market. For the breeding majority of the farmers opt for natural service as the availability of quality semen is very limited. In the case of, Kangayam the average size cattle holding was found as 2-3 with the average milk yield of 4-6 lit/day. The farmers expressed that, this cattle has unique advantages of raising in low external input system with grazing, resistance to diseases & adverse climate conditions and almost all the farmers in the study area are consuming only indigenous cattle milk and crossbred animals was exclusively kept for economic returns through the sale of milk. Further, it was found that there is a huge demand for Kangayam cattle milk in the nearest towns and sold at the rate of ₹ 80-100/lit. In the case of Umblachery breed, it was found that the majority of the farmers rear this breed exclusively for its dung quality, which is very ideal for organic/natural farming in the study area. The average size cattle holding was found as 6 as the majority of the farmers holding upto 10 hectares of cultivable land, with the average milk yield of 2.5 lit/day. The Umblachery Breeders Association formed in the year 2004 is actively involving in its conservation and promotion of entrepreneurs through training in making different products from animal waste viz, Panchgavya, cosmetics/curing & pain reliever and had established an exclusive market for its milk, ghee and other by-products and sold at premium price. In the case of Pulikulam breed, popularly known as 'Jallikattu' (bull taming game) breed, which is primarily being used for the sport purpose and also for 'Herding', where individual farmers' herd were joined, moved together and stationed in the cultivable lands over a night for its dung and urine, which is the major source livelihood for the rearers. Due to the increased awareness among the general public about its importance for 'Jallikattu', now it becomes an incentive for rearing this breed, which also ensures the effective system of breeding. Further, the offsprings of the bull winning the jallikattu will be valued high and there is a huge demand for male calf among the farmers and the general public, which makes them to feel proud and prestigious in up-keeping these cattle.

Major challenges faced by indigenous cattle owners

The major challenge often posed towards indigenous cattle breed was its low milk productivity than the crossbreds. In most of the cases, indigenous cattle breeds are well-adapted to their resource-specific regions and are maintained with low external input system. However, in better resource system/or a commercial system of dairying crossbreds outperforms in terms of higher economic benefits in a short span of time. Hence, a major challenge is to enhance the productivity of the indigenous cattle and improved adoption of improved management practices by the farmers. The major challenges faced by indigenous cattle rearers include:

- Low genetic potential of indigenous cattle breeds
- Non availability of breed specific semen and AI infrastructure in the breeding tracts
- Non-availability of community grazing land/access to forest area/CPRs
- Inadequate supply of green fodder and other feed resources during the scarcity period
- Lack of financial support, incentives and promotional schemes from the government
- Lack of exclusive market for indigenous cattle milk and products for a premium price
- Non coverage under cattle insurance scheme
- Lack of credit support from financial institutions
- Lack of awareness and training regarding preparations of various products from dung and urine
- Inadequate data based on indigenous cattle
- Lack of farmers participatory breed conservation programmes
- Lack of recognition to local breeds and nomadic herds

Prospects of indigenous cattle farming

Indian history is strongly bonded with cattle, especially cow for its milk, as the milk is not just a drink, it is an elixir for almost every individual from child to an elderly person. Further, the cattle have become an integral part of the agricultural production system by converting the farm waste/ by-products into high-value milk for human beings and other critical inputs like dung and urine back to rejuvenate soil health in the same agricultural production system. In this regard, the local breed, suited to the locality has played an immense role in securing the nutritional as well as economic security of the farmers. Since ancient times, different breeds were developed in different parts of the subcontinent by selecting the best animals for preferred traits, such as their milking capacity, draught power, feeding requirements, the capacity to adapt to local weather, immunity, *etc.*

The purity of such breeds was maintained with great discipline and wisdom in each geographical pocket known as a breeding tract. Over time, unfortunately, this social rigour was lost. Indiscriminate mating between different breeds and inferior animals within the same breed resulted in a high number of cattle of poor genetic quality. This is due to the fact that, these local breeds were neglected for a long time in characterization, conservation and planned breeding programme. Sustainable livestock production is dependent in proper utilization of our local genetic resources and hence, the developmental strategy of indigenous cattle must emphasize upon the purpose of rearing, its suitability to agro-ecosystem and affordability of the rearers. The indigenous cattle, apart from its milk, it is valued for its other by-products made out of cattle dung and urine and further, form as a nucleus in organic farming. The following are the distinguishable characteristic features of indigenous cattle farming which offers enormous potential benefits:

- Increasing demand for indigenous cattle milk and other products like Dahi and Ghee
- Importance to Organic farming - Panchagavya, Gobar and Gomutra
- Potential enterprises activities through - preparation of various products from cow dung and urine
- Highly sustainable in local agro-climatic conditions
- Environment-friendly cow based farming

Successful Entrepreneurs: few cases from the field

- Shri. Puravi Muthusamy, Muthur, Tirupur Distt, Tamil Nadu
- 35 Indigenous cattle (Kangayam, Gir, Red Sindhi) and 11 acres of land
- KOVARSHINI -Panchakavya and herbal care products –started in 2009 - with 30 lakh investment - cottage level
- Cow dung and Urine as a base products -12 products – cosmetics/ curing & pain reliever, Panchgavya, Ghee, etc.
- Got trained from Govigyan Anusandhan Kendra, Nagpur
- Monthly net income around ₹ One lakh

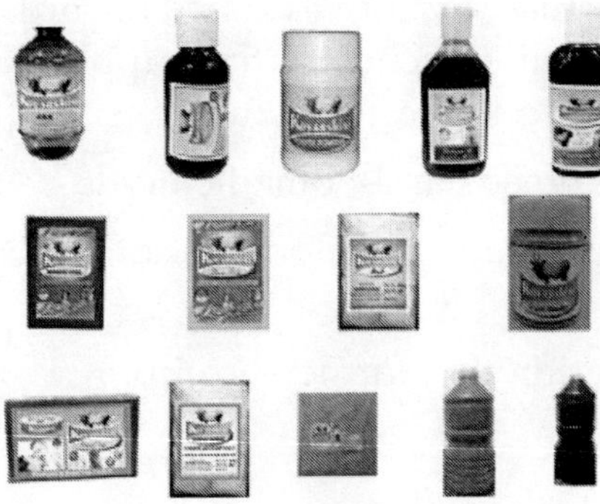

Korkai Umblacherry Goshala

- Breders Association -Started 2004
- Shri. B.Janakiraman -President
- Owns 80 cattle, maintains >100 years
- Exclusive market
- Prepares different by-products

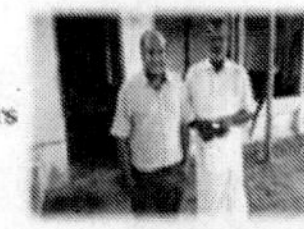

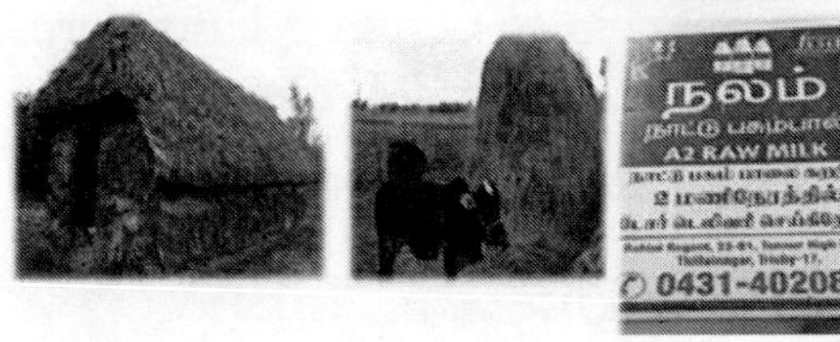

Herding

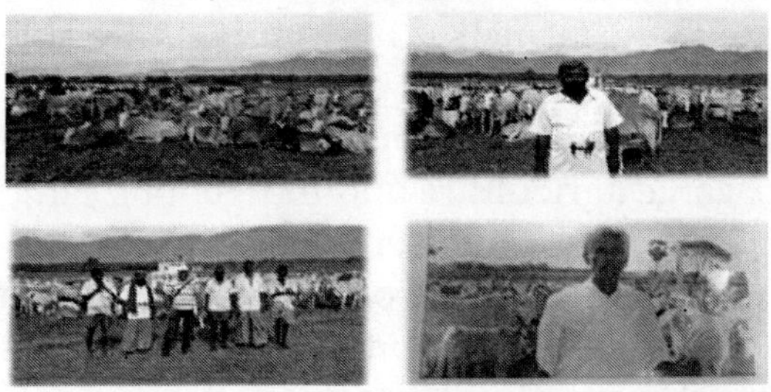

Gokulam Goshala

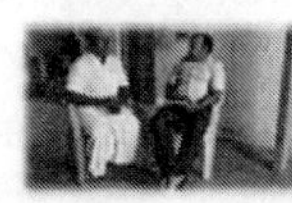

- Shri. Sivaraman, Thottakacheri village, Thiruvarur, Tamil Nadu
- 100 Indigenous cattle (Kangayam, Gir, Red sindhi, malnad gidda, deoni, umblachery etc) and 10 acres of land
- Nandhini -Panchakavya and herbal care products -2014 - with 10 lakh investment - cottage level
- Cow dung and Urine as a base products
- 9 products - cosmetics/curing & pain reliever, Panchgavya, Ghee etc
- Got trained from Govigyan Anusandhan Kendra, Nagpur
- Monthly net income around Rs.50,000

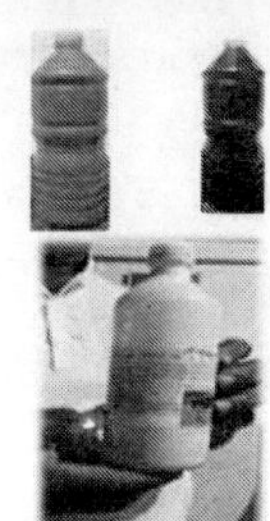

Policy implications

- Selective breeding of quality indigenous cows in their breeding tracts; using these improved breeds to upgrade the non-descript stock
- Promotion of Farmers participatory breed conservation programme
- An assured supply of quality input supply like semen, feed and fodder resources
- Exclusive market for the indigenous cattle milk and other by-products with a premium price

- Specific programmes/special schemes/incentives aimed towards indigenous cattle farming-free animal scheme, the supply of screened bull/credit, insurance, vaccination coverage
- Recognition of indigenous cattle breeds and nomadic herds
- Access to Grazing land, forest areas and development of CPRs for grazing & water sources
- Training on by-products preparation to a farmers group

Conclusion

Indigenous cattle play an important role in providing subsidiary income and nutritional security to the farmers. These animals are able to sustain on low external input system and are climate resilient and adapted to the local conditions. There is a strong growing concern among the farmers towards organic agriculture and indigenous cattle farming due to changing priorities of the end user-consumers. Hence, the prerequisite for sustainable development of indigenous cattle farming includes: Promotion of Farmers participatory breed conservation programme, assured supply of breed-specific semen, development of feed resources/grazing lands through community participation, and provision for the exclusive market with a premium price, which will subsequently promote indigenous cattle farming in our country.

References

19th Livestock Census, (2012). Department of Animal Husbandry, Dairying & Fisheries, Ministry of Agriculture, Government of India.

Concept paper on Rashtriya Gokul Mission, (2014). Department of Animal Husbandry, Dairying and Fisheries, Ministry of Agriculture, Government of India.

http://www.planningcommission.nic.in/aboutus/committee/

K.P. Ramesha. "Significance of Animal Genetic Resources in the Modern IPR Era vis-a-vis Climate Change Scenario-Indian Perspective". Compendium of ICAR Short course on "Recent Advances in Animal Genetic Resources Conservation Technologies and its Significance in the Modern IPR Era vis-a-vis Climate Change Scenario, held at SRS, NDRI during 18-27 July, 2013.

Chapter 15

Unique Physico-chemical Qualities of Indigenous Cattle Milk

Laxmana Naik, N., Surendra Nath B., K.P. Ramesha and P. Heartwin Amaladhas

Introduction

Milk and milk products are the main constituents of the human daily diet for all age group people since the times of domestication. Milk of some animals, especially cow, buffalo and goat, etc., are used for human consumption, either as such or in the form of a range of dairy products. Milk and milk products provide an important array of nutrients including high-quality protein, fat, carbohydrates and many other essential nutrients in the almost ideal proportion, which are necessary for health. It never ceases to amaze that, hundreds of ingredients are produced from the single source 'milk'. These ingredients are used in thousands of applications (Pe Boer, 2014). Since the time of Ayurvedic medicine, there is an evidence of special mention with respect to the use of milk & milk products derived from indegineous cow (*Bos indicus*) or desi cow. Scientific evidence also suggests that milk from zebu (humped) cattle has several advantages over the milk of exotic cattle. In general, consumer prefers to use desi cow milk over the crossbred and other bovine milk owing to the rich taste, flavour and palatability. Scientifically, this quality perception can be ascribed to the uniqueness of desi cow milk composition and constituents with respect to an array of essential fatty acids, essential amino acids, vitamins, mineral, antioxidants and antimicrobial substances. Due to these reasons, the indigenous cow milk and milk products are in great demand. Therefore, in this chapter, an effort was made to highlight the unique physico-chemical qualities of indigenous cattle milk in comparisons to exotic and buffalo milk.

Milk-The Nature's "*Perfect Food*"

Milk is one of the highly evolved secretions of mammary glands of mammals and the most perfect food for their infants. Milk is a complex biological fluid composed of water, lipids, carbohydrates, proteins, minerals, pigments, enzymes, vitamins, and a long list of essential valuable constituents. Characteristics of these constituents and associated benefits have made milk an important part of the human diet. There are innumerable health benefits credited to milk and milk products. Milk is an important source of nutrients including high-quality proteins, fat, carbohydrates and many other nutrients necessary for health in almost ideal proportion. Hence, milk from dairy cows is considered nature's single most complete food (O'Mahony, 1988). American nutrition authority has heralded milk as "nature's perfect food" as "indispensable" as the "most complete food" (DuPuis, 2002). Milk and milk products are widely used as components of many food products. The contributions of milk consist of excellent nutritive value, unique flavour, desirable texture and a widely accepted "natural" image. In many instances, the success of the product in the marketplace is significantly enhanced by incorporation of traditional functional ingredients familiar to the consumer. Thus, milk and milk-based dairy ingredients provide a consumer-friendly label on packaged foods.

Milk can be defined in various ways. Chemically speaking, milk is a complex fluid in which milk fat is present in the form of an emulsion, protein and some mineral matters are in the colloidal state and lactose with some minerals and soluble proteins are present in the form of a true solution. Biologically, milk is the lacteal secretion; practically free from colostrum, obtained by the complete milking of one or more healthy milking animal. From a physiological standpoint, milk is the secretion of the normally functioning mammary gland of the females of all mammals, which is produced for some time, following parturition for the nourishment of the young of the species during the initial period of growth. In terms of physical chemistry, milk is an opaque, whitish fluid of multi-disperse phases. The true solution contains lactose, vitamins, acids, enzymes, and some inorganic salts. The colloidal phase contains casein, calcium phosphate, and globular proteins. Fat exists in the form of an oil-in-water type of emulsion, with fat globules varying from 0.1 to 22 μm in diameter. From a nutritive standpoint, milk is defined as the "most nearly perfect food." In legal terms, milk may be defined as the lacteal secretion, practically free from colostrum, obtained by the complete milking of one or more healthy animals. According to the Food Safety Standard Authority of India (FSSAI) rules, cow milk should contain not less than 8.3% of milk solids-not-fat and not less than 3.2% of milk fat. The gross composition of milk significantly varies and these are influenced by the breed and species of the milk animals, feeding pattern, lactation period, the interval between milkings as well as health and age of the animals. In addition, changes to the milk occur, after it is harvested and before it is processed, which may affect its processibility.

Milk of some animals, especially cow, buffalo, goat and sheep are used for human consumption, either as such or in the form of a range of dairy products. A great variety of milk and milk products, shelf-stable dairy beverages and dairy foods are exclusively prepared from milk. Apart from these, pharmaceutical, personal care, infant food, bakery products, confections, soup, savoury snacks, feed, and non-food applications are based on milk in one or other form. Milk has fully accepted as essential and extraordinary importance, it has contrast medicine. It can be a natural nutraceutical with extra health benefits in addition to the basic nutritional value (Hajare, 2017). Many kinds of literature reports on mining of milk for the health-promoting constituents (peptides, fatty acids, milk sugar and minerals). Increasing sophistication in advancement and refinement of qualitative and quantitative techniques has focused attention to append new molecular components to this list with special attention to trace components of potential health significance (Naik *et al.*, 2013).

From time immemorial, it is worldwide wisdom that fresh raw milk is the best and complete diet, our tradition called cow's milk as Ambrosia (*Amrut* in Vedas). Traditional information about desi cow milk is complex, and it is not clear, most of the reported findings are pertaining to western breed milk composition. There is a need for exhaustive research on the elucidation of indigenous cattle milk unique quality and explore the true health benefits. In this milieu, research teams consisting of the above authors are working on the "Elucidation of physicochemical quality and neutraceutical properties of Deoni and Malnad Gidda indigenous cattle milk and ghee".

Genetic Resources Diversity of Indigenous Cattle Breeds in India

India is a mega biodiversity hub of animal genetic resources and contributed richly to the international livestock gene pool and improvement of animal production in the world. The vast and varied forms of Indian animal genetic resources are playing a crucial role in providing livestock security to rural masses. Seventy-nine per cent of about 300 million bovines in India are indigenous. India has been home to 43 indigenous breeds of cattle, in addition to the vast cattle population, which comes under the nondescript category. There are 3 major types of cattle breeds as per their utility: (i) Milch breeds–Sahiwal, Gir, Rathi and Red Sindhi (few animals only at organized farms); (ii) Draft breeds–Amritmahal, Bachaur, Bargur, Dangi, Hallikar, Kangayam, Kenkatha, Kherigarh, Khillari, Malvi, Nagori,Nimari, Ponwar, Umblachery, Red Kandhari and Siri, and (iii) Dual-purpose breeds – Deoni, Gaolao, Haryana, Kankrej, Krishna Valley, Mewati, Ongole and Tharparkar. Vechur and Punganur are the dwarf breeds. The population of some breeds like Nagori, Hariana, Ponwar, Kherigarh, Mewati, Hallikar, etc. is declining mainly due to mechanization of agriculture. In addition to these, there exist some stable populations in different regions that significantly contribute to the food and agriculture production of that region. These are Alambadi, Binjharpuri, Ghumsuri, Pullikulam, Kumauni, Ladakhi, Malnad Gidda, Mampati, Manipari, Motu, Red Purnea, Shahabadi, Gangatiri, ThoTho, and Tarai. There are no wild relatives of cattle in India (Country Report on Animal Genetic Resources of India, Govt. of India, 2007).

Unique Features of Indigenous Cow

Indigenous cattle (*Bos indicus*) differ from *Bos taurus* cattle found in Europe and North American in morphological characters. A prominent hump, a long face, upright horns, drooping ears, a dewlap and slender legs characterize the indigenous breeds. Indigenous cattle have a lower basal metabolic rate, better capacity for heat dissipation through cutaneous evaporation and thus, adaptation to tropical heat and resistance to diseases specially the tick-borne diseases than *Taurus* cattle. Indigenous breeds are well known for heat tolerance, hardiness and ability to survive and perform even under stressful conditions and low input regimes. They can recognize their owners even after the lapse of considerable time (Ramesha, 2003). Different breeds of indigenous cattle (*Bos indicus*) were evolved over centuries to suit to different agro-ecological situations (Ramesha and Dixit, 2017).

Desi cow in India (Indigenous cow) has always been widely respected and worshipped. The hump in desi cow has a specific vein called surya ketu nadi, which is absent in non-vedic cows. This nadi (*vein*) absorbs all the energies and radiation from the sun, moon, and all luminaries from the universe and puts them in cow-like milk, dung, ghee (clarified butter). Desi cow has vein connected to sun passing through her backbone sebum gland, it has believed to that this nadi absorbs the medicinal essence from the sun and improves the nutritional value of milk (Hajare, 2017).

Indigenous Cow Milk: Unique physico-chemical Qualities

In the food pyramid, milk and dairy foods form an important component of a healthy balanced diet. Milk consumption has been called a marker for an overall healthy diet because of its association with increased nutrient intake. In India, a separate market segment is emerging as a desi cow milk and milk products category. The indigenous cattle (83.4%) population contributes 47% of cow milk (Desi cow milk, A2 milk), while crossbred (16.6%) contributes 53% of cow milk (a mixture of A1 and A2 milk). Cow-milk has always been a part of the Indian diet. Its spiritual and nutritional values have been known to our ancestors since time immemorial. Our ancient Ayurvedic texts describe the Indian cow-milk as possessing a sweet taste, cooling in nature, highly nutritive, a tonic for our vital organs, easily digestible, and whose consumption promotes immunity and longevity (http://saveindiancows.org/benefits-of-drinking-pure-desi-cow-milk/).

Research finding on A1 and A2 type milk reveal that majority of the native cow are also of A2 type and are shown to be of homozygous A2A2 for beta casein genotype (Naik *et al.*, 2013, Ramesha *et al.*, 2016). Investigations conducted at ICAR-National Bureau of Animal Genetic Resource revealed that 618 animals were screened from different breeds of Zebu cattle (indigenous breeds). The allelic frequency for A2 was found to be 98.7%, while for A1 it was 1.3%. Malnad Gidda and Kherigarh, both these breeds expressed A1A2 and A2A2 genotype, rest of all screened animals are of A2A2 genotype (Mishra *et al.*, 2009).

A traditional herder from the Gawli community, who conserves the rare Gaolao breed of cattle from Wardha district in Maharashtra, reports that the milk from Gaolao cows is thicker and sweeter, and good for children's growth. "It makes very tasty khowa and the ghee has richer fragrance and taste". Taking the example of the Gaolao breed, there is a lot of traditional knowledge surrounding the milk quality and its connection with the various kinds of wild grasses consumed by Gaolao, which has traditionally been an open grazing breed." One of these grasses, known locally as paonya, it is said to impart greater taste and nutrition to milk and ghee. Ghee from cows fed on paonya grass, known as *paonya chya toop*, is regarded as the best quality ghee in these areas. (http://www.downtoearth.org.in/blog/the-deshi-cow-milk-jinx-45095).

The Vechur cattle is a rare breed of *Bos indicus* cattle named after the village Vechoor in Kottayam district of the state of Kerala in India. With an average length of 124 cm and height of 87 cm, it is the smallest cattle breed in the world according to the Guinness Book of Records (2012) and is valued for the larger amount of milk it produces relative to the amount of food it requires. The milk is believed to have medicinal qualities and easy digestibility due to smaller fat globule size (Thirupathy and Iype, 1997). The protein component of the Vechur cow's milk has an improved antimicrobial property (Shashidharan *et al.*, 2011). As per recent findings, the anti-bacterial property of the lactoferrin protein present in the Vechur cow milk is more than that of the antibiotic ampicillin. The Ghee produced from Vechur cow's milk is also famous for its high medicinal values.

A recent study shows that the presence of gold in cow urine and milk in Gir cow, therefore, there is something unique in the desi cow. Traditionally Indian cows are reared mainly based on grazing, which results in milk production with low in saturated fatty acids, cow fed on green grass produce conjugated linoleic acid (CLA) rich milk. The indigenous cow milk has high levels of CLA, a vital health promoter. Rich sources of carotenoids, which imparts a yellow colour to the indigenous cow milk, which is good for eyes. Vitamins D and B_{12}, anti-microbial substances viz. lactoferrin, lysozyme, and immunoglobulins levels are also high. The content of lactoferrin, a well-known anti-microbial and antiviral protein is higher in desi cow milk as compared to crossbred cow and buffalo milk. The cholesterol content in desi cow milk fat is lower than buffalo and exotic cow milk. The fatty acids found in it are more beneficial to human health. Because of these reasons, the medicinal properties of milk of indigenous cow milk are widely found application in Ayurvedic system of medicine.

Milk from cows grazed or fed on fresh forage, especially from species-rich grasslands or forage legumes, has a considerably higher ratio of unsaturated to saturated fatty acids and a higher content of nutritionally beneficial trans-fatty acids (e.g. CLA, vaccenic acid) than milk from cows fed silage or hay (Kalac and Samkova, 2010). In a pilot study, Deoni milk chemical composition and physicochemical properties were investigated by Kumar (2004). A higher proportion of long-chain saturated fatty acids, conjugated linoleic acid, and Vitamin E as compared to exotic cattle were reported in Deoni milk fat (Smitha, 2004). Unsaturated fatty acid (USFA) level was 40.46% and Tocopherols level was 36.05-38.5µg/g fat.

Sowmya (2016) collected milk samples from 85 *Deoni* breed cow and reported that average values for milk fat and SNF were 4.8±0.05 and 9.50±0.02, respectively. Arjun (2017) reported that pooled *Deoni* milk samples fat and SNF were in the range of 4.1-4.9 % and 9.09-9.68 %, respectively. Thimmesha *et al.*, (2018), reported that the average pH value of *Deoni* and *Malnad Gidda* cow milk was 6.59±0.014, and 6.64±0.013, respectively. The average fat globule size for *Deoni* and *Malnad Gidda* cow milk was 3.7 and 3.2µ, respectively. The specific gravity (at 20°C) of *Deoni* and *Malnad Gidda* cow milk was 1.031±0.0018 and 1.029±0.0013, respectively. The relative viscosity (cP) was 1.76±0.06 and 1.53±0.04, respectively for *Deoni* and *Malnad Gidda* cow milk. The specific heat was found to be 3.818, and 3.850 J/kgK, and electrical conductivity was found to be 3.25 and 3.7 mili Siemens/cm, respectively for *Deoni* and *Malnad Gidda* cow milk.

According to the report of Ramesha *et al.* (2015), Malnad Gidda cow milk is having a characteristic flavour, colour and odour. Possibilities of excretion of these medicinal and aromatic chemical compounds and their metabolites from feed to milk might have increased the nutritional and therapeutic value of Malnad Gidda cow milk. Malnad Gidda milk has significantly higher beneficial anti-microbial substance lactoferrin (225.20 ± 31.40, mg/L) as compared to Deoni (99.95 ± 7.48 mg/L), crossbred cattle (ranged 42.59 to 91.89 mg/L) and Murrah buffaloes (ranged 11.75 to 47.13 µg/ml) (Ramesha *et al.*, 2014). Malnad Gidda milk has the lowest somatic cell score as compared to milk from other breeds reared in the same region. There is a huge demand for Malnad Gidda cow milk and other products particularly ghee due to a preference for usage in ayurvedic medicine preparation.

Important differences in the milk of indigenous cow, exotic cow and buffalo milk qualities are compiled based on various reports and presented in Table below.

Table 1: Important differences between the milk of Desi, Exotic breeds and Buffalo

Sl. No	Characteristics	Indigenous cow milk	Exotic cow milk	Buffalo milk	Remarks (Benefits/Adverse effects)
1.	Colour	Creamy yellow	Creamy yellow	White	Carotenoids benefits in decreasing the risk of disease, particularly certain cancers and eye disease.
2.	Taste and Flavour	+++++	+++	++++	Consumer prefers to buy milk which is rich in taste, pleasantly sweet and clean flavor.
3.	Consistency	Thick	Thinner	Thick	Rich Consistency and palatability.
4.	Calorific Value	+++	++	++++	Higher fat in buffalo milk results in more calorific value.
5.	Keeping quality	++++	+++	+++	Naturally produced preservative compounds are more in Indigenous milk than other milk.
6.	Curd strength	+++	+++	++	Soft curd helps in better Digestibility and easy assimilation of nutrients.
7.	Fat globule size (Average)	3.4 μ	4.5 μ	5.67μ	Smaller size, better the assimilation than the larger globule. More yellow and softer texture butter is desirable and widely acceptable.
8.	Casein-Type	A2 Milk (A2 type casein)	A1 and A2 type milk (A1 as well as A2 type casein)	A2 Milk (A2 type casein)	A2 milk is good for milk. A1 milk is reported to be associated with various diseases in individuals having leaky gut syndrome. In babies where mucous membrane is yet to be developed. The difference in A1 and A2 beta-casein is the amino acid histidine in A1 and proline in A2 milk at position 67. On digestion of A1 casein, BCM7 (beta-casomorphin 7) is released but not in A2 casein. Several reports (based on animal studies) available on the adverse effect BCM7 on human health-related to Type 1 diabetes, Heart disease, Sudden Infant Death Syndrome, autism, digestive disorders, neurodegenerative disorders, intolerance, allergies, autoimmune conditions. Animal studies have shown digestion of A1 milk promotes the formation of oxidized LDL, a marker of heart disease.
9.	Conjugated Linoleic Acid (CLA) Content	High	Low	Medium to high	CLA -vital health promoter. Helps in good cardiac health, disease resistance and boosts brain development in children. CLA has anti-carcinogenic properties. Immuno-modulating and antiatherogenic properties.
10.	Saturated Fats, Short-chain Fatty acids	Low (Good for health)	High	low	The low rate of fat hydrolysis, better keeping quality and long shelf-life.

11.	Unsaturated Fats,	High (Good for health)	Low	High	The more grain in a cows diet, the more unbalanced ration of EFA (Essential Fatty Acids) in her milk i.e Milk produced from pasture-reared cows are best for health and sold at a higher price in developed countries.
12.	Omega3: Omega 6 ratio near one	The ratio is almost 1:1	Omega 3 is low & Omega 6 is high (2 to 3 times higher) depends on the type of diet	The ratio is near to 1:1 reared on green fodder	Green Fodder is the best and cheapest option for Balanced Omega3 Omega 6, low Saturated fat content of milk.
14.	Carotenoids (Lutein, Zeaxanthin and Beta Carotene)	High (30 μg/g in grazing animal)	Very low	Very low (0.25 to 0.48 μg/g)	Cows reared based on grazing or grass-fed cows produce milk with high carotenoids. This imparts yellowish in colour to milk. Lutein, Zeaxanthin and Beta Carotene are most important antioxidants associated with healthy eyes and postpones AMD (age-related macular degeneration).
15.	Vitamin D	High	Low	Low/Nil	Stallfed (due to low sunshine exposure)- have poor Vitamin D in milk. Indian cows graze that effect in high sunshine exposure resulting in higher Vitamin D in milk.
16.	Antibiotic residues	Generally nil	High due to various treatments	Low	As Exotic cattle suffer more from mastitis, foot-related diseases and reproductive problems high level of antibiotics are generally used, resulting in antibiotic residues in milk.
17.	Lactoferrin	Highest	Low	Low	An immune defensive protein possess Antimicrobial and antiviral property
18.	Somatic cells	Low	High	Low	Higher the somatic cell, inferior the quality milk.
19.	Mineral profile	High	Low	Medium to high	Minerals are required in large quantities by the rapidly growing neonate for bone growth and development of soft tissues

Conclusion

Since the time of Ayurvedic medicine, evidence shows that milk and milk products derived from desi cow is preferred. At the present context also consumer prefers to use desi cow milk over the crossbred cow or other milk, owing to the rich taste, flavour and palatability. Because of this reason in the last few years, desi cow milk market segment is emerging and has created a separate market segment.

Scientific evidence also suggests that milk from desi cattle has several advantages over the milk of exotic cattle. The overall quality and consumer acceptability are governed by many parameters, as discussed above and hence, it may not be appropriate to conclude solely by the extent of variation and concentration of the particular constituent. Scientific study both at micro and macro level for many such compounds, which are responsible for enhancing the neutraceutical and medicinal value of desi cow milk are yet to be established. Such a study-in addition to providing valuable information on the quality of milk will also help the farmers maintaining the indigenous cattle to realize the value for milk from indigenous breeds.

References

Arjuna V.M. (2017). Development and Validation of Formulae for the Estimation of Solids-not- fat and Total Solids in Cow and Buffalo Milk. *MSc Thesis*, ICAR-NDRI, SRS, Bengalore-30.

Country report on animal genetic resources of India, (2007). Department of animal husbandry & dairying ministry of agriculture government of India. ftp://ftp.fao.org/docrep/fao/010/a1250e/annexes/countryreports/india.pdf

De Boer, R. (2014). *From milk by-products to milk ingredients: upgrading the cycle*. John Wiley & Sons.

DuPuis, E.M. (2002). Why Milk. *In:* Nature's Perfect Food: how milk became America's Drink. NYU Press.

Guinness World Records, (2012). "Smallest cow (Height)"Retrieved January 6, 2012.

Hajare, R. (2017). A1 Milk Needle in a Haystack. *J Tradit Med Clin Natur.* 6: e133

http://saveindiancows.org/benefits-of-drinking-pure-desi-cow-milk

http://www.downtoearth.org.in/blog/the-deshi-cow-milk-jinx-45095

http://www.idfa.org/news-views/media-kits/milk/importance-of-milk-in-diet.

Kalac, P. & Samkova, E. (2010). The effects of feeding various forages on fatty acid composition of bovine milk fat: A review. *Czech Journal of Animal Science*, 55(12): 521-537.

Kumar Gaurav (2004). A Study on the physico-chemical properties and chemical composition of milk from Deoni breed of cattle. MSc Thesis, ICAR-NDRI, SRS, Bengalore-30.

Mishra, B.P., Mukesh, M., Prakash, B., Sodhi, M., Kapila, R., Kishore, A. & Bujarbaruah, K.M. (2009). Status of milk protein, b-casein variants among Indian milch animals. *Indian J Anim Sci*, 79: 722-5.

Naik L., Mann B., Bajaj, R. Sangwan R.B. and Sharma R. (2013). Process optimization for the production of Whey protein hydrolysates: Adopting response surface methodology. *International Journal of Peptide Research and Therapeutics*, 19(3): 231-237.

Naik Laxmana, Kiran Lata, Rajan Sharma, Y.S. Rajput and Abhishek (2013). Health implications, Science behind A1 and A2 Milk, Food and Beverage News: Aug. 16-31: 27-30.

O'Mahony, F. (1988). Rural dairy technology: Experiences in Ethiopia. International Livestock Centre for Africa, Addis Ababa, Ethiopia. ILCA Manual No. 4, Dairy Technology Unit, 3 & 8 pp.

Ramesha, K.P., Singh, A.P., Isloor, S., Basavaraju, M., Akhila Rao, Divya, P., Ananthraj, A.and Varalakshmi, S. (2014). Identification of Genetic Variants of Lactoferrin Gene and its Association with Lactoferrin Content and Somatic Cell Count in Bos Indicus Cattle. News letter, ICAR-NDRI, Karnal, 19(2): 9.

Ramesha, K.P. (2003). Indigenous cattle and their role in this millennium. Swadeshi Pathrike, 28-32.

Ramesha, K.P. (2016). Livestock and Poultry Bio-resources of Karnataka and their future prospects for access benefit sharing mechanism. *In*: Tradable Bio-Resources in Karnataka, 133-169.

Ramesha, K.P. and Dixit, P.K. (2017). Indigenous cattle-Crucial for human health, sustainable agriculture and environment. TCS Koppa, Sahakara Sarige Rajat Mahotsav, 66-72.

Shashidharan, A., Singh, R., Bhasker, S. & Mohankumar, C. (2011). Physicochemical characterization and functional site analysis of lactoferrin gene of Vechur cow. *Bioinformation*, 6(7): 275.

Smitha (2004). Physico-chemical characteristics of milk lipids of Deoni breed of Cattle. *MSc Thesis*, ICAR-NDRI, SRS, Bengalore-30.

Sowmya H.S. (2016). Development of a formula for estimation of solids not fat in milk and its validation- A pilot study. *MSc Thesis*, ICAR-NDRI, SRS, Bengalore-30.

Thimmesha, Laxmana Naik, Surendra Nath., Heartwin P. Amaladhas, K. P Ramesha, Ramakrishna Prasad and Deena Joseph. (2018). Elucidation of Deoni and Malnad Gidda Cattle milk quality"

E-PosterQA-13, at 46th Indian Dairy Association conference held at Kochi during 8-10 Feb., 2018.

Thirupathy Venkatachalapathy, R., & Iype S. (1997). Fat globule size and distribution in milk and iodine value of milk fat of Vechur cattle of Kerala. *Indian journal of animal sciences*, 67(10): 910-912.

□□□

Chapter 16

Indigenous Cattle Waste: A Valuable Bio-Resource

Mukund A. Kataktalware, Menon Rekha R., S. Jeyakumar and K.P. Ramesha

In India, livestock has been an integral constituent of the agricultural based rural economy, providing energy for crop production in terms of draught power and organic manure, and in turn, drawing their own energy requirements from crop by-products and residues. The advances in biochemical and mechanical technologies, however, have undermined the synergy between livestock and crops. Livestock is now more valued as a source of food and contribute over one-fourth to the agricultural gross domestic product and engage about 9 per cent of the agricultural labour force. Similarly, Cow (*Bos indicus*) urine, one of the ingredients in *panchagawya,* is believed to have therapeutic value and since ages are being used for the treatment of several diseases under the traditional system of medicine. However, in recent years, attention has also shifted to the negative impact of livestock waste on the environment and their effects on water quality, soil deterioration, air pollution, and the rural-urban interface. Land application of excessive quantities of nutrients is subject to surface runoff and leaching that may contaminate ground or surface water. If managed properly, manure can be a valuable bio-resource for a farm. It can be a source of nutrients for crop production and can improve soil quality. The goal of animal waste management should be to make the best use of the nutrients in manure while protecting natural resources. Indigenous bovines are robust and resilient and are particularly suited to the agro-climatic conditions of their respective breeding tracts and are gifted with unique qualities of heat tolerance, resistance to various diseases and the ability to thrive under extreme climatic stress and less than optimal nutrition. Ignoring the lifetime production and other numerous contributions, repeatedly indigenous cattle are compared with high yielding exotic/

crossbred cattle (Kataktalware *et al.*, 2017). Against this background, it is high time to reveal multifarious uses of not only milk but also of by-products of indigenous cattle, which would re-establish its 'real economic value'.

Uniqueness of Indigenous Cattle Dung

Since ages cow dung has been used as organic fertilizer in Indian sub-continent. Before the advent of inorganic fertilisers, it was the major source of plant nutrients added to the soil. Similarly, Indigenous cow (*Bos indicus*) urine one of the ingredients in *panchagawya* is believed to have therapeutic value and is being used for the treatment of several diseases under the traditional system of medicine. Normally, the composition of cow dung is about 80% water which supports a matrix of undigested plant material that is rich in nutrients, micro-organisms, and their by-products. Cow dung microflora contains an abundant number of bacilli, lactobacilli and cocci and some identified and unidentified fungi and yeasts (Muhammad and Amusa, 2003). The lower part of the gut of the cow contains various micro-organisms including *Lactobacillus plantarum, Lactobacillus casei, Lactobacillus acidophilus, B. subtilis, Enterococcus diacetylactis,* Bifido bacterium and yeasts (commonly *Saccharomyces cerevisiae*) having probiotic activity (Ware *et al.*, 1988). There are several pieces of evidence to show that fresh cow dung and cow urine are anti-fungal and antiseptic in nature (Nene, 2003), which might be due to secretion of antimicrobial metabolites by cow dung microflora. The comparison of chemical composition of dung of *desi* and crossbred cows which were fed common basal diet revealed that there was no difference in the organic matter, nitrogen and manganese contents in the two types of cow dung, contents of calcium, phosphorus, zinc and copper were higher by 10.8, 8.0, 84.1 and 21.7 per cent in the dung of *desi* cows than that of crossbred cows (Garg and Mudgal, 2007). The addition of cow dung increases the mineral status of soil, enhances the resistance of plant against pests and diseases; stimulate plant growth (Naskar *et al.*, 2003) and other beneficial activities such as sulphur oxidation and phosphorus solubilization (Sharma and Singh, 2015).

Indian Scenario

In 2010, Federation of Indian Chambers of Commerce and Industry has undertaken the "Resource Assessment Study for Agro-Industrial and Livestock Wastes-India" and reported that on an average a cattle farm produces manure in a range of 15 to 100 MT/ day depending upon number of animals and waste water generated was found to be in a range of 15,000 L/day to 100 m^3/ day, while other types of wastes like fodder and hay, fat and grease may lie in the range of 25 kg/day to 1500 kg/day (Anonymous, 2010). They reported that most common manure management practice is aerobic treatment like composting (40%), followed by dumping in pits (40%) resulting in methane emissions and sun-dried manure (20%) which is used as fuel for cooking and heating purposes. An insignificant amount of waste water is generated at the farm level from animal washings and cleaning the farms. Some farms have established anaerobic digesters with biogas collection system, however, because of various reasons, most farms are currently non-operational. Organisations encounter a multitude of problems in erection and operation of methane recovery and utilization units because of lack of technical know-how at a farm level. Some of the technical problems reported to be faced by during operation are improper mixing of cow dung, less production of biogas in winter season, maintenance problem, problem in slurry management, leakages, insufficient gas formation, inadequacies in design, gas pressure regulation, methane gas collection, storage, and utilization, irreparable damages caused due to improper handling (Anonymous, 2010). There is a need to undertake systematic research to address the above-mentioned problems so that the potential of such a valuable bio-resource is utilized efficiently.

Fertilizer

The indiscriminate use of chemical fertilisers has led to the deterioration of soil health causing erosion in its productivity. It warrants re-storation of the soil health by using farmyard manure (FYM) as an organic fertilizer. To compensate a lower content of NPK in the dung, it is suggested to enrich the same with certain botanicals/ herbs, microbes/ fungi, which would enhance its potential as bio-fertilizer (Kataktalware *et al.*, 2017). If the dung of indigenous cattle is collected and processed locally, it can be put to better use. The co-operative model of milk sector can very well be applied for collection, processing, and distribution of value-added manure. The livestock owners could be offered a remunerative price for the unutilized dung and the end-user will be benefitted by improved soil fertility. The collateral benefits of the model are environmental protection, savings on subsidy and sustainable agriculture. Similarly, the collection, processing and distribution can open up new job opportunities. The economies of scale would help in reducing the cost of installation of the capital-intensive system used for electricity generation from biogas. The electricity generated can be made available to local communities and surplus can be supplied to the grid. The digestate can be suitably fortified to enhance its potential as bio-fertilizer, suitably packed and marketed. The slurry, which contains minor nutrients, also can very be applied to the agriculture field.

Energy

Waste-to-energy schemes that generate revenue from the energy produced and may provide fertiliser as a valuable by-product offer an alternative and environmentally acceptable means of disposal of waste. The caloric value of manure depends on the composition of the waste and moisture content. With the concern over future energy shortages and increasing costs of conventional fuels and electricity derived from them, much interest is directed towards using anaerobic digestion as a source of renewable energy while providing acceptable waste management. Biogas (CH_4 plus CO_2) formed during anaerobic digestion is approximately 65% CH_4 and has a heat of combustion of 21.7 MJ/m3 (20°C, 1 atm). The resulting sludge is much less odorous (stabilized) than raw manure and contains the nutrients (N, P, and K) that were in the original manure (Smith *et al.*, 1979). The produced gas can be utilized as fuel for cooking, lighting, electricity generation, etc. Two biogas plants of 85 m^3/day capacity are said to be suited for electricity generation in a small village of 100 households (Belsare *et al.*, 2007). In recent years, with the objective of disposal of various organic wastes in an environment-friendly manner, the interest in setting up biogas plants has increased. There has also been a growing interest in using the biogas slurry as suitable manure for organic farming by substituting the inorganic fertilizer with biogas slurry. The initial investments for such projects are considered high, when compared to the power generating projects based on conventional fuels. The purpose of these projects, however, is not to generate energy alone but to dispose off wastes and therefore, the investments can be justified. With indigenization of technology, advancement of processes for the generation of biogas and more number of plants, the initial investment is expected to reduce significantly (Gautam, 2006).

Medicinal Use

Recently, indigenous cow urine has caught the attention of policymakers, the scientific community and a lot of research work is going on exploring its unique medicinal properties. Banga *et al.* (2005) reported that the bio-enhancing/immuno-enhancing properties of cow urine exist only in the urine of indigenous cow and not in the urine of other species like buffalo, goat or not even in crossbred cows. Similarly, Jarald *et al.* (2008) evaluated cow urine and its distillate for anti-oxidant and anti-microbial activities and reported that comparatively fresh cow urine was found to be better than its distillate in exhibiting activities tested, supporting the claim of traditional practitioners. Such scientific validations would open new markets for indigenous cow urine, which, if tapped properly in collaboration with NGO's, Gaushalas, *Mathas* may go a long way in conservation of indigenous cow and income generation for resource-poor farmers (Kataktalware *et al.*, 2010).

Conclusion

Animal waste, if properly handled and processed, could be converted into a tangible asset. With proper policy support, it has the potential to generate additional income for milk producers. It is hoped that in long-term, it will help in the conservation of indigenous cattle and sustainable agriculture.

References

Anonymous, (2010). Resource assessment study for agro-industrial and livestock wastes–India. Federation of Indian Chambers of Commerce and Industry. (www.methanetomarkets.org/.../292_5_ficci_resource_assess_jan_10.pdf DOA 20/10/10).

Anonymous, (2017). Annual Report 2016-17, Department of Animal Husbandry, Dairying & Fisheries, Government of India.

Azevedo, J. and P.R. Stout, (1974). Farm animal manures: An overview of their role in the agricultural environment. California Agr. Exp. Sta. Ext. Service Manual 44. p 109.

Banga, R.K., Singhal, L.K. and Chauhan, R.S. (2005). Cow urine and immuno-modulation: An update on cowpathy. *International Journal of Cow Science* 1(2): (http://www.indianjournals.com/ijor.aspx?target=ijor:ijcs&volume=1&issue=2&article=002 DOA 20/10/10)

Belsare, V.P., Kapdi, S.S. and Varshneya, M.C. (2007). Electricity generation using cattle dung- An overview. In: National Symposium on Recent Trends in Policy Initiatives and Technological Interventions for Rural Prosperity in Small Holder Livestock Production System organized by Sri Venkateswara Veterinary University, Tirupati and Indian Society of Animal Production and Management at College of Veterinary Science, Tirupati during 20-22, June 2007. Pp: 65-67.

Garg, A.K and Mudgal, V. (2007). Organic and mineral composition of *Gomeya* (cow dung) from *Desi* and crossbred cows – A comparative study. International Journal of Cow Science. 3: (http://www.indianjournals.com/ijor.aspx?target=ijor:ijcs&volume=3&issue=1and2&article=003 DOA 20/10/10)

Gautam, H.C. (2006). India Country Profile on Animal Waste Management for Methane to Markets. (www.methanetomarkets.org/documents/ag_cap_india.pdf DOA 20/10/10)

Jarald, E., Edwin, S., Tiwari, V., Garg, R. and Toppo, E. (2008). Antioxidant and anti-microbial activities of cow urine. *Global Journal of Pharmacology* 2(2): 20-22.

Kataktalware, M.A., Das, D.N. and Ramesha, K.P. (2010). Livestock waste management: environmental protection and value addition. In: Advances in Dairy Production: Precision output, environment and trade. Edt by Dr. B. Srinivas and Dr. A. Obi Reddy. Published by SRS, NDRI (ICAR, New Delhi), Bangalore-30. P: 146-160.

Kataktalware, M.A., Menon, R.R., Jeyakumar, S. and Ramesha, K.P. (2017). Utilization of indigenous cattle manure. In: Souvenir of National Seminar on Strategies for Enhancing Productivity of Indigneous Cattle organized by Alumni Association, SRS, iCAR-NDRI, at ICAR-NDRI, SRS, Bengaluru on 1st July, 2017. Pp: 57-60.

Muhammad and Amusa. *In vitro* inhibition of growth of some seedling blight inducing pathogens by compost inhibiting microbes. *Afr. J. Biotechnol.* 2003; 2(6): 161–164.

Naskar Sethuraman S.K., Ray P Rc. Sprouting in plants by cow dung slurry. Validation of Indigenous Technical Knowledge in Agriculture Extension. Indian Council of Agricultural Research. 2003; 197-201.

Nene Y.L. (2003). Crop diseases management practices in ancient, medieval, and premodern India. *Asian Agri. Hist.* 7(3): 185–201.

Sharma, B. and Singh, M. (2015). Isolation and characterization of bacteria from cow dung of desi cow breed on different morpho-biochemical parameters in Dehradun, Uttarakhand, India. *International Journal of Advances in Pharmacy, Biology and Chemistry*, 4(2): 276-281.

Ware Fungsin D.R., Read P.L., Manfredi E.T. (1988). Lactation performance of two large dairy herds fed Lactobacillus acidophilus strain BT 1386. *J. Dairy Sci.* 71: 219–222.

□□□

Chapter 17

Intellectual Property Rights: Its Strategic Use in Livestock Sector for Value Extraction

K.P. Ramesha and Mukund A. Kataktalware

India is home to 184 indigenous breeds of livestock and poultry with unique traits, which include 43 for cattle, 16 for buffalo, 34 for goat, 43 for sheep, 7 for horses & ponies, 9 for camel, 8 for pig, 2 for donkey, 1 for yak, 19 for chicken, 1 for duck and 1 for geese. Besides recognised breeds, there are populations of livestock and poultry in various geographical locations with unique traits. About 70 per cent of milk is produced by marginal and small farmers owning 2-4 animals. The different production systems like zero input-low output, low input-moderate output, intensive input-high output are characteristics of the dairy production system in India (Ramesha and Divya, 2013). The milk productivity of indigenous cow, crossbred cow, buffalo and goat is only 3.41, 7.33, 5.76 and 0.45 kg/day in the year 2015-16, respectively, which needs to be improved substantially.

Indigenous livestock have evolved over a long time in the diverse, stressful, tropical environment with adaptive traits. This situation enables them to live and engender in these conditions. The milk productivity of indigenous cattle and buffaloes could be enhanced substantially by the adoption of various modern technologies for selection and faster multiplication of genetically superior germplasm and adoption of improved animal management. The future development of the livestock sector depends on the adoption of new and innovative production and processing technologies, and proper market tie-ups. Diversification and high-value produce will add new dimensions to this sector. A paradigm shift is required in livestock sector from a production orientation to quality and cost orientation in the WTO era (Ramesha 2011), which could be achieved by technological advancement for which innovation is the key. In the present knowledge-based global economy, protection of intellectual property (IP) is critical for technology development and diffusion in all fields including the livestock sector (Ramesha *et al.*, 2010). In the last few decades, rapid progress has been made in animal breeding and genetics. Animal breeders and geneticist have started protecting their intellectual property, which has alarmed livestock keepers, other scientists and the public. Intellectual Property protection has increased with the sequencing of the genome, production of transgenic and cloned animals.

At the international level, Convention on Biological Diversity (CBD) of United Nations and Trade-Related Aspects of Intellectual Property (TRIPs) Agreement of World Trade Organization are the two major agreements governing access and rights over genetic resources. As India is a signatory to both CBD and TRIPs, there is a need to assess the IPR issues in animal breeding with a global perspective and also, evaluate the options for the typical livestock production situation existing in the country.

Convention on Biological Diversity (CBD)

The CBD is a legally binding international instrument, which recognizes the sovereignty of nations over their genetic resources, including the capacity to establish conditions of access by other nations and a fair/equitable sharing of benefits from the use of such resources. As such, the animal genetic resources have not been the objects of much specific consideration within the CBD, and no consideration has been given to arrangements that meet the special nature and distinctive features of the livestock sector. The main objectives of the Indian Biological Diversity Act (2002) was to comply with CBD are conservation of biological diversity, sustainable use of its components and fair and equitable sharing of the benefits arising out of the use of biological resources and knowledge. In India, patent applications have to disclose the source of genetic material and associated Traditional Knowledge (TK) in relevant cases. TK has the potential of being translated into commercial benefits by providing leads for the development of useful products and processes. Hence, creators and holders of TK must get a share of benefit. It might be worth giving attention to the need and possibility for developing a "clearing-house" mechanism to operate at the Deptt. of Animal Husbandry and to the possibility of conducting an IPR audit.

Trade-Related Aspects of Intellectual Property Rights (TRIPs)

Under TRIPS Article 27.3, members must provide various forms of intellectual property, many of which are relevant to animal genetic resources and animal products, including indications of geographical origins, trademark, trade secrets and patents. It provides that member countries must grant patents on all products and processes, except that they may exclude from patenting the plants, animals and essentially biological processes, other than microbiological ones. Provision is made for plant variety protection under patents or a *sui generis* system, or a combination of both. There is no comparable system for animals. Animal patenting, even in countries, where it is permitted, is so far largely a phenomenon of medical and pharmaceutical research, rather than of livestock agriculture, though this may change with the introduction of transgenic animals. Patents and trade secrets are relevant to animal biotechnology research and development. In the animal sector contractual arrangements, trade secrets, trademarks and patents have relevance.

IPR regime and Animal Genetic Resources

Intellectual Property (IP) is a category of property that confers rights over intangible creations of human intellect. IPRs are legal and institutional devices to protect creations of the mind. India is a signatory to both Convention on Biological Diversity (CBD) and TRIPs Agreement and also ratified Global Plan of Action on Animal Genetic Resources (AnGR) adopted in September 2007, therefore, it is obligatory for India to develop suitable legislation to protect and improve livestock biodiversity and associated traditional knowledge. TRIPs agreement provides effective protection to the following 7 forms of IPRs:

1. Patents/protection of plant varieties and plant breeder's rights
2. Copyrights and related rights
3. Trademarks
4. Industrial designs
5. Layout Designs (topographies) of Integrated Circuits
6. Geographical Indications
7. Trade Secrets.

IPR are largely territorial in nature except for copyright, which is global in nature. These rights have to be renewed from time-to-time for keeping them in force except in case of copyright and trade secrets.

Patents

A patent represents a legal monopoly granted by a country's government to an inventor, permitting the patent owner to prohibit anyone else from making, using or selling this invention for a specific period of time (presently 20 years). The aim of a patent system is to encourage economic and technological development by rewarding intellectual creativity. IP system safeguards the rights of an inventor in his invention/intellectual richness while benefitting the end-users and society as a whole. The purpose of the patent system is to protect inventions and encourage fair competition in the field of technology so as to transform inventions or creations into real and productive forces. Intellectual property is an important and effective policy instrument to a wide range of socio-economic and technological concern. It is to be remembered that the possession of a patent not only confers certain monopoly rights and privileges of the patented article but certain obligations and duties also. Commercialization of IP-enabled technologies is an absolute necessity to transfer valuable technologies, developed in the Institute laboratories to the society for the greater benefit of mankind.

The various national and regional patent systems are receiving and granting patents in the field of the livestock sector, while policies and regulations concerning the sectors are being articulated as a topic for discussion in the CBD and FAO forum. Intellectual property laws have the potential to alter the existing legal conditions for competition and investments in the livestock field and needs, therefore, a higher level of awareness among policy-makers, breeders, scientists and farmers. Patenting of living organisms is a contentious issue among the WTO member states. Under TRIPS Article 27.3, members must provide various forms of intellectual property, many of which are relevant to the livestock sector, including indications of geographical origins, trademark, trade secrets, patents and copyright. Provision is made for plant variety protection under patents or a *sui generis* system, or a combination of both. There is no comparable system for animals. Biotechnology firms are interested in patenting processes and genes used in animal breeding as such. The patenting of broad traits like increased milk yield or broad claims on genes/animals may lead to monoculture and monopoly, which would result in suffering to the pastoralists, small and marginal farmers. With the advent of genetic engineering and multilateral IPR agreements, a new era of gene hunting has started. Researchers, innovators and companies have now started to protect their intellectual property in the livestock sector.

Patenting in living forms

Patenting of life forms is the most controversial aspect even among WTO members. Judgement in the Diamond vs. Chakrabarthy case in US Supreme Court in 1980 had a lot of impacts worldwide in patenting of living organisms. The question, in this case, was whether one particular genetically engineered bacterium could be patented; the US Supreme Court responded with the all-encompassing statement that "anything under the sun that is made by man" is patentable. This judgement had a major impact on the legal situation throughout the world because it laid the groundwork for altering the basic principle that patent protection is not available in the field of food production (Rothschild *et al.*, 2004). The first patent on animals of higher biological classes than micro-organisms was granted in the Oncomouse case, where a mouse was genetically modified for use as a laboratory research animal. Since the area of patenting of farm animals is new, the number of relevant court and panel decisions is very limited, which increases the relevance of using practice from laboratory animals in this area even though the sectors are different. A modified animal gene is eligible for patent protection in most of the countries.

Scope for patenting in livestock sector arises from the fact that, though any living form that has existed in nature does not qualify for a patent, anything created by human ingenuity and application of human intellect, if 'new' and 'non-obvious', is in principle patentable. Different technologies in the livestock enterprises can receive protection by breeder's rights, patents, trademarks, geographic appellations, copyright and industrial design depending upon the nature of technology; they will receive protection by one or a combination of different IPRs (Sunitha Ninan *et al.,* 2005).

IPRs with Special Reference to the livestock sector

Biotechnology is providing the capability to produce novel genetically modified organisms (plants, microorganisms, fishes and animals), which are commercially valuable and industrially useful.

As per the Indian Patents Act (IPA), plants & animals in whole or any part thereof other than GMO and essentially biological processes for production or propagation of plants and animals are not patentable. However, whole organisms like transgenics, produced with human intervention are patentable in India. Under the TRIPs agreement, farmers have to get legal protection for their traditional knowledge (including that of livestock) via patents or by an effective *sui generis* system or by both. National Bureau of Animal Genetic Resources (NBAGR) have been identified as a nodal institute to register and document valuable animal genetic resources respectively by ICAR. The registration system will bring elite germplasm into the public domain to promote its use in research, however, the system does not have any legal backing.

In the livestock sector, patents have been granted for gene sequences with a utility such as genetic markers. A New Zealand company, Agmark, has claimed a patent on the "Booroola" gene, which regulates the ovulation rate in sheep. The Booroola gene can be traced back to Bengal sheep, which were imported from Kolkata and crossed with Merinos (Köhler-Rollefson, 2005). The patent covers animals that are produced in a breeding programme, in which the DNA test has been used, but not those animals that carry the gene naturally. The open question is whether the patent also covers the offspring of the animals that have been tested for the presence of the gene. Another notable patent application is one by Monsanto for a series of twelve patents on pig breeding. One of the first conflicts in quantitative animal breeding resulted from a patent entitled "Method of Bovine Herd Management" granted to the Cornell Research Foundation (Cornell University) in the USA in 1994 and Canada, in 1998. The invention is for the "test-day model" and includes the gathering of data, mathematical treatment and the use of the data by dairy producers (Rothschild *et al.*, 2003; Scholtz and Mamabolo, 2006). The novelty and non-obviousness of the patent have been seriously questioned. The practices of gathering, manipulating and using data by dairy producers have existed for nearly 100 years (Schaeffer, 2002). In South Africa, these principles have been in use since 1917. The patent, therefore, claims rights to a practice that has been in public knowledge for a long time. The novel idea within the patent is the specific mathematical model and procedures that were developed for the analysis of test day yields.

In the European Union and some other countries, patents can also be granted on normal animals, which have merely been subjected to certain techniques like a gene diagnosis, or a process for determining the animal's sex. The European Patent Office granted a patent on Dolly the cloned sheep to the Roslin Institute in Edinburgh (patent application EP 849 990) in 2001. The US Company XY Inc. was in 2005 granted patent EP 1257168, which covers a method for selecting sperms by sex for the artificial insemination of mammals. The first European patent on genetically manipulated dairy cows was granted in 2007. Under patent number EP 1330552 "inventors" from Belgium and New Zealand claim processes for breeding cows, which give more milk or milk with altered constituents. The cows are produced either by marker-assisted breeding and bred normally or by having more milk genes additionally incorporated into their genome. Hungary is one of the few countries that grant patent protection for animal breeds (WIPO, 1995). The Bulgarian Law for Protection of New Plant Varieties and Animal Breeds have been enforced since 1996. In terms of the patentability of higher life forms, such as animals and fishes, they are not treated any differently by the Australian Patent Office from the way in which lower lifeforms are treated. The East African Boran cattle breed has also been patented in Australia (Scholtz and Mamabolo, 2006). The practice in New Zealand is similar to that of the Australian Patent Office. In general, patents to animals are allowed in Japan. In contrast to these countries, animals (whether transgenic or otherwise) are not patentable in countries, such as Argentina, Brazil and China (Blattman *et al.*, 2002) and India (Ramesha *et al.*, 2010, 2011).

IPR issues in the field of living organisms

Before the availability of modern biotechnological tools, inventions based on living organisms were treated as natural phenomena i.e. discoveries and were not patentable.

There are concerns in the area of

- **The limits of patentability:** In biotechnology research, many times it is difficult to distinguish between invention and discovery. The isolation of a gene from its natural environment and the identification of its function render the gene and its sequence an invention for patenting purposes in some countries.

- **Patenting of "enabling technologies":** This issue is of great importance, as it has an impact on access to these technologies by the animal research system in general.
- **The multiplicity of patents required to develop a livestock product:** Developments in modern livestock biotechnology require the use of several processes and products, which in most cases will be subject to patent protection. For example, producing transgenic livestock involves several processes, such as identification of gene of interest, inserting the gene at appropriate stage, to check the gene incorporation, to study the gene expression, checking the animals having inserted genes, etc.
- **Patents on specific genes usually extend to the GM organisms into which the genes are inserted, thus bringing the entire organism under patent protection:** This question has raised considerable debate. Eventual financial revenues are granted to the patent holder, without compensating the developers of the original plant/animal variety.
- **Concentration of the IP in the hands of few MNCs:** In the modern biotechnology era, there is danger of animal genetic material from biodiversity rich countries being exploited by others including large international companies. Another important element is that a small number of multinational companies (MNCs) dominate livestock biotechnology field. Existence of strong IPRs, and the fact that the rights over the technologies and products are often owned by MNCs, might lead to (increased) dependence by developing country farmers on MNCs and developed countries. With the development of modern biotechnology, there is possibility that indigenous breeds/varieties may be genetically altered and the new variety/breed may later be substituted for the original breed/variety, from which it was developed.
- **Patenting of indigenous livestock genetic resources:** Patents can and have been issued to companies from developed countries over genetic material from developing countries. In some cases, the lack of appropriate mechanisms for sharing of benefits has generated considerable controversy.

In recent years, there is a study increase in the number of patent applications filled in animal and fishery sector. A good number of patent applications has been filed by various ICAR institutes and agricultural and allied sector universities in the field of animal, veterinary and fishery sector.

Trademarks

Trademarks are signs or symbols registered by a manufacturer/ producer or merchant to identify goods and services. A trademark can be a word, phrase, symbol, design, or a combination thereof, example: Cadalmin™. Many countries also recognize "collective marks" and "certification marks". Collective Marks are a sign which distinguishes the origin of a product, method of production and distinctive characteristics of goods or services. A collective mark may be owned by an institution or co-operative or a public entity and used by members of the organization, example- "AAA". Certification marks - like CE (European conformity) and The Good-housekeeping seal of approval–"certify" that products or services meet a particular standard of quality, regional origin or the like, even though the products may come from various unrelated companies. Certification marks- are a sign used to denote the origin of the product that meets set standards and specifications. Certification marks are similar to collective marks except that users of certification marks should not necessarily be members of the organization that owns the mark, example- "Wool Mark". Genetic material *per se* cannot be protected or covered by a trademark. A trademark can be a useful value addition tool. The trademark can improve the value of a product. For example, semen straws, dairy products, from a reputed company with a trademark may fetch a higher price.

Geographical Indications

Geographical Indications (GIs) are signs or expressions used on goods to indicate that a product or service originates in a country/ region or specific place, where a given quality, reputation or another characteristic of the good is essentially attributable to its geographical origin. Both Trademarks and GIs are used to identify the products and help to create wealth and improve the competitive position of businesses. A Trademark puts emphasis on the producer or a manufacturer of a product whereas a GI highlights the geographical origin of a product and the characteristics derived from it. GI does not protect the breed or genetic material *per se* but adds commercial value to the animals of a breed reared in a particular region. They may be used as a value addition mechanism. Geographical indications prevent all others, other than the producers of goods from the original region from using that particular geographical indication incorrectly as a trademark for other products than those from the area. Registration of Darjeeling tea, cultivated in 87 designated locations in the Darjeeling Region helped to prevent misappropriation and improved marketing position and income.

Ethiopia produces some of the finest coffee in the world but gained very little as there was a problem of misappropriation, but the filing of trademark applications in 36 countries and securing protection in 30 countries helped to differentiate the Ethiopian fine coffee from the coffee of other countries. This helped to build confidence and improve the bargaining position of coffee producers and exporters from Ethiopia and increased the price of Ethiopian coffee and income of coffee producers, which resulted in a positive improvement in the living standard of farmers. In France, Bresse breed of chicken is produced in the Bresse geographical area only, as defined by law under a protected designation of origin (Verrier *et al.*, 2005) and sold at 50-60 per cent higher price. Similarly, to save the Sambucana sheep from extinction, a consortium was set up and a special brand name for guaranteed Sambucana meat was set up in Italy. Roquefort cheese can be made only from the milk of the Lacaune sheep breed. Chilika buffaloes with typical curd made from its milk, and Banni, Dharwari buffaloes with typically flavoured milk products are other examples, which could be considered for protection (Ramesha, 2008). Under GI, the production system is characterized by natural conditions and a production system unique for that area. There is scope for utilizing GI based on unique characteristics of products produced from a breed in a geographical area due to natural conditions and unique production system.

Trade Secrets

Trade Secrets (in certain circumstances and jurisdictions called know-how) provide protection against unauthorized disclosure or use of confidential information (of a technical or commercial nature). To be protected as a trade secret, the intellectual property must, of course, be kept secret, and must also confer some sort of commercial advantage to the holder. Enforcement of IP rights for trade secrets is possible, when a competitor has misappropriated and/or stolen the trade secret. Trade secrets are important in animal and fish breeding, where commercial breeders want to keep their nucleus stock and the pedigree information (and other information) away from their competitors.

A point often raised is when one should file for a patent or maintain the information as a trade secret. What is important to note is that patents and trade secrets are not in conflict with each other but are complimentary IP assets. Depending upon the nature of the know-how; or the invention, the organization may choose to either file a patent or to continue to hold as a trade secret.

Need of the hour

IP protection of technology should be to the mutual advantage of the producers and users of technology in a manner conducive to the social and economic welfare of the society. The development of a legally binding "International Framework on Animal Genetic Resources" is, therefore, becoming a matter of urgency.

Epilogue

Identification of genes for unique characteristics in native livestock will go long way not only in the advancement of science but also pave way for patenting of gene sequences for these traits. The IPR and other legal instruments influencing knowledge intensity of livestock sector is complex and are greatly influenced by knowledge generation and management. Our country with a large number of well-trained veterinary, animal science personnel and large livestock resource should develop a suitable environment for innovation by appropriate Science and Technology policy as well as IP policy, which is critical for economic development of the sector, which is concerned with livelihood security of a huge number of rural folk. We should make use of all the available flexibilities in TRIPs in the IP system to suit the specific needs particularly with respect to traditional knowledge.

References

Blattman, J., McCann, J., Bodking, C. & Naumsoka, J. (2002). Global intellectual property: International developments in animal patents. In: Intellectual Property Rights in Animal Breeding and Genetics. Eds. Rothschild, M.F. & Newman, S., CABI Publishing, New York. pp. 63-84.

Köhler-Rollefson, (2005). Building an International Legal Framework on Animal Genetic Resources, Can it help the dry lands and food-insecure countries League for Pastoral Peoples?

Ramesha, K.P. and Divya, P. (2013). Recent advances in animal genetics for enhancing dairy animal productivity in India. Paper presented in the 42nd Dairy Industry Conference, 12-14th December, 2013, Chennai, India.

Ramesha, K.P. and Jayaraj Rao, K. (2013). New trends in Indian Dairy Sector. CommodityIndia.com. 13(12): 23-26.

Ramesha K.P., Pourouchottamane R and Bhattacharya, M. (2007). Role of indigenous livestock genetic resources in the era of modern Intellectual Property Rights. Indian Dairyman, 59(11): 39-45.

Ramesha, K.P., Sadana, D.K. and Goswami, S.L. (2010). Modern IPR Regime-a boon or a bane for livestock biodiversity. Indian Dairyman, 62(8): 74-79.

Ramesha, K.P. (2011). Intellectual Property Rights Regime for livestock agriculture in India - present status and future prospects. JIPR. 16(2): 154-162.

Rothschild, M.F., Plastow, G. & Newman, S. (2003). Patenting in animal breeding and genetics, in A. Rosati (ed.) *WAAP Book of the Year 2003*. Wageningen Press, for World Association for Animal Production (WAAP).

Schaeffer, L.R. (2002). Dairy cattle test day models: A case study. *In: Intellectual Property Rights in Animal Breeding and Genetics*. Eds. Rothschild, M.F. & Newman, S., CABI Publishing, New York. pp. 233-246.

Scholtz, M.M. Mamabolo, J. (2006). A developing country perspective on recent developments in animal breeders and intellectual property rights. African J. of Biotechnology, 36(5): 22-25.

Verrier, E., Tixier-Boichard, M., Bernigaud, R. and Naves, M. (2005). Conservation and value of local livestock breeds: usefulness of niche products and/or adaptation to specific environments. Animal Genetic Resources Information. 36: 21–31.

WIPO (1995). Database of Intellectual Property, Hungary Law No. XXXIII of 1995 on the Protection of Inventions by Patents, Pp 1-35.

❑❑❑

Chapter 18

IP Management in Agriculture with Special Reference to Livestock Sector

Letha Devi G. and Mukund A. Kataktalware

In the present knowledge-based world economy protection of intellectual property (IP) and knowledge management are critical for technology development and diffusion in all fields including the livestock sector. A paradigm shift is required in livestock sector from a production orientation to quality and cost orientation in the WTO era. The knowledge-based technological revolution in livestock sector helped dominant players to corner the benefits at the cost of smallholders, particularly in poultry and pig industry in many parts of the world. IPRs give the creator the right to prevent others from making unauthorized use of their property for a limited period. There are various types of IPRs. Only some are relevant to the livestock sector. These include patents, trademarks, trade secrets and geographical indications. Each of these forms of IPR has different requirements and grants different legal status.

Patents

Patents grant an exclusive right to prohibit others from using an invention for commercial purposes. Patents are given, if an invention fulfills the criteria of:

- Being new compared with what was previously known (prior art).
- Involving an inventive or non-obvious step, and being capable of industrial application.

Patents can be granted on products and on processes. Patents are "territorial rights" and only granted and effective in the countries that they have been applied for. So, if a patent has been granted in Australia, then the invention is patent-protected only in that country and not elsewhere. Basically, each country has its own national patent law in which it defines what can be patented and what not. However, in Europe, there is only one institution dealing with patent applications, the European Patent Office (EPO) in Munich.

The World Intellectual Property Organization (WIPO) accepts applications for patents that it then forwards to all other countries. WIPO is also seeking to harmonize patent law worldwide by establishing a substantive patent treaty that will be globally effective.

All member countries of the World Trade Organization (WTO) have to comply with the TRIPS (Trade Related Intellectual Property Rights) Agreement, which sets certain minimum standards for intellectual property protection.

In the livestock sector, patents have been granted for gene sequences in connection with genetic markers. A New Zealand company, Agmark, has claimed a patent on the "Booroola" gene, which regulates the ovulation rate in sheep. The patent covers animals that are produced in a breeding programme in which the DNA test has been used, but not those animals that carry the gene naturally. The open question is whether the patent also covers the offspring of the animals that have been tested for the presence of the gene. Another notable patent application is one by Monsanto for a series of twelve patents on pig breeding. It is currently pending at WIPO.

The rationale of patents is that they should provide incentives for innovation, research and development. But it is doubtful whether they would really fulfill this purpose in the animal breeding sector, and there is worry that they would, in fact, inhibit use of animal genetic resources by researchers, breeders, and farmers.

In addition, it is rather questionable whether much of the kind of research that is patentable, such as cloning and genetic engineering, is actually supportive of the sustainable management of animal genetic resources, and in line with animal welfare requirements.

Trademarks

Trademarks are distinctive signs, such as symbols, letter, shapes or names that identify the producer of a product and protect its associated reputation. Well-known examples include the Coca-Cola lettering, McDonald's "golden arches", and "Kentucky Fried Chicken".

Genetic material itself cannot be trademarked, but a specific type of product from a specific breed can be. For instance, there is a registered trademark for certified Angus beef. Organic producer associations also have obtained registered trademarks for their goods, such as Demeter, Bioland, Naturland, *etc.*

Trade Secrets

Trade secrets consist of commercially valuable information that is kept secret from competitors. As long as they remain secret, trade secrets are protected by laws, which prevent acquisition by commercially unfair means and unauthorized disclosure. Trade secrets do not establish an exclusive right over a genetic resource but have been used with great success by genetics companies in the poultry sector and in hybrid pig breeding. These companies go to great length to keep their nucleus stock and information about pedigrees out of reach of competitors. They also make use of biological locks to enforce their trade secrets, for instance, by releasing one-day old chicks only of the same sex to prevent others from using them for breeding.

Geographical Indications

Geographical Indications identify the specific area of origin of a product, and the associated qualities, production process, reputation, and other characteristics. They do not protect the genetic resource but can add value to products of a particular breed in a particular region. Examples from Europe include Parmigiano-Reggiano cheese, Feta cheese, Bresaola of Valtellina, and Prosciutto di Parma ham. Roquefort cheese can be made only from the milk of the Lacaune sheep breed. Examples from developing countries are Karoo lamb (South Africa) and Chos Malal goat meat (Argentina). There is strong evidence from both developed and developing countries that origin-based marketing in which control over production processes remains with the livestock keepers can empower them versus corporate interests and provide greater earning power.

Sui Generis System

The term *sui generis*is used in the TRIPS Agreement in connection with the protection of plant varieties. It means that an IPR law of its own kind - adapted to the specific needs of the crop sector - can be developed as an alternative to patenting.

There have also been efforts to develop a sui generis system for traditional knowledge by WIPO. The possibility of crafting a sui generis system for the protection of animal genetic resources, tailored to the requirements of the livestock sector has also been discussed. On one hand, such a sui generis system could provide the context for establishing Livestock Keepers' Rights (see below); on the other hand, there seems to be a basic incompatibility between traditional knowledge and IPRs.

Livestock Keepers' Rights

The concept of Livestock Keepers' Rights has been developed over a period of almost seven years in a series of livestock keepers' and pastoralists' meetings on three continents. The cornerstones of this concept include:

- Recognition of livestock-keepers as creators of breeds and custodians of animal genetic resources.
- Recognition of the dependency of the sustainable use of traditional breeds on the conservation of their ecosystems.
- Recognition of traditional breeds as collective property, products of indigenous knowledge and cultural expression.
- The right of the livestock keepers to make breeding decisions.
- The right of livestock keepers to participate in policy-making processes on issues relating to animal genetic resources.
- Support for training and capacity building of livestock-keepers in the provision of services along the food chain.

Some governments, including India and African countries, support the concept of Livestock Keepers' Rights, but other governments regard them as unexplored legal or political ideas. Some experts believe that Livestock Keepers' Rights could conflict with patents on genes.

Patenting Activities in Veterinary Sciences

India is a huge country of animal biodiversity contributing a large quantity of milk, meat, egg, draught power, fibre, manure, etc. generating rural employment. In order to improve the sustainable productivity of livestock in India, it is absolutely necessary to increase technological inventions and their protection. Animal scientists have now started to protect their intellectual property and these protective measures have alarmed other scientists and the public. The diversification in Indian agriculture was also noticeable during the period 2005 to 2012 as dairy products and animal husbandry registered 19.0 and 5.78 times increase in patenting activity over the period 1995-2004, besides development of new plants and processes (10.87 times) and horticulture and cultivation forestry rising (5.87 times). In India, the number of patent grants has increased significantly in all the fields of agricultural sciences particularly in the fields of transgenic, agro-chemicals and animal vaccines after the introduction of patent reforms in 2005 and accumulation of the applications during the transit period (Kandpal *et al.*, 2015).

Maximum percentage of patent applications were filed in biocides, pest repellents or attractants and plant growth regulators (60%), followed by new plants or processes for obtaining them (9.35%), animal husbandry, silk rearing or breeding new animal breeds (7.48%) and (5.91%) horticulture, cultivation, forestry. The challenge for biodiversity-rich countries is to guard against bio-piracy of their indigenous animal genetic resources and to safeguard technologies that they have been using. Another concern is the export of genetic material to countries that did not ratify the Convention on Biodiversity (Scholtz and Mamabolo, 2006). More than 80 patents have been filed by the scientist researchers working in the area of veterinary science research at Indian Veterinary Research Institute, Izzatnagar. Moreover, a total of 11 patents has been granted for the livestock technologies developed by the institute (www.ivri.nic.in). However, more than 25 patents have been filed during the last 5 years by the National Dairy Research Institute, Karnal. The institute has developed the various technologies in the research area of dairy science.

Some of the technologies developed and commercialized in the recent past in the field of livestock farming by ICAR institutes Area specific mineral mixture for different agro – MINKAM-UT is ecological zones (example- a quality product researched & developed by Indian Veterinary Research Institute, Izzatnagar & licensed technology transferred by National Research Development Corporation, New Delhi (Patented) fortified with Vitamins (A, E & D3 & Probiotics). 'Crystoscope' is a field tool used for determining the optimum time for fertile insemination or for timely heat detection in cattle and buffalo, "Olinall" herbal ointment for the treatment of chronic skin ailment, FMD vaccine, complete feed block technology developed using locally available unconventional feed, cost-effective detoxification technologies for oil.

Conclusion

The patenting in veterinary sciences is meagre might be due to non-consideration of parameters like biological processes, methods and animals in whole or any part thereof is not eligible for patenting. The patent reformation in the year 2005, allowed patenting of product and process in all fields of science including veterinary science, which has accelerated the activity of patenting in India. The need and importance of patenting of technology are being recognized in India, an increasing trend, development of financial agencies and technology appraisal agencies for patenting in veterinary sciences needs to be strengthened. Issues of protecting intellectual property in veterinary science should receive urgent attention at national and international level particularly from developing countries like India. The effects of IPRs on animal genetic resources on genetic diversity, genetic improvement and the livelihoods of livestock-keepers have scarcely been analysed, but are in urgent need of exploration. The customary right of livestock-keepers to breed their animals, which has been the driver of livestock biodiversity, may be under threat - unless specific national and international legal frameworks are developed.

References

Ingrassia, A., D. Manzella, and E. Martyniuk, (2005). The legal framework for the management of animal genetic resources. FAO Legislative Study 89, Rome.

Kandpal, A., Bhooshan, N. and Pal, S. (2015). Recent Trend in Patenting Activity in India and its Implications for Agriculture. Agricultural Economics Research Review, 28(1): 139-146.

Tvedt, M.W., S.J. Hiemstra, A. Drucker, N. Louwaars and K. Oldenbroek, (2007). Legal aspects of exchange, use and conservation of animal genetic resources. Fridtjof Nansen Institute, Lysaker, Norway.

Scholtz M.M. and Mamabolo J. (2006). A developing country perspective on recent developments in animal breeders and intellectual property rights. *South African Journal of Animal Science*, 36(5): 22-25.

❑❑❑

Chapter 19

Technology Management and Entrepreneurship Development in Animal Husbandry Sector

P. Sethuraman Sivakumar

Indian agriculture is the second largest in the world in terms of its total output. The agriculture contributes 14.4% of national GDP and employs about 48.9% of the total workforce (Ministry of Finance, Government of India; Economic Survey, 2010-11). In the post-economic liberalisation era, Indian agriculture has slowly transformed as an industrial sector, with a focus on maximising its economic value. The Agricultural Universities belong to the state and central agencies have contributed significantly in maximising output in agriculture thereby enhancing livelihood security of the farmers and other stakeholders. In recent years, there has been a significant structural change in agriculture, with an increasing focus on the entrepreneurial advantage of the traditional profession. In line with this trend, there is a growing interest among universities in pursuing commercial applications of research, including new venture creation. This transition has led to several questions on the role of universities and associated research institutions in creating and sustaining entrepreneurship in their respective regions.

1. Agricultural entrepreneurship

Entrepreneurship is the process of creating something new with value by devoting time and effort, assuming the accompanying financial, psychic and social risks and uncertainties; and receiving the resulting rewards of monetary and personal satisfaction. The purpose of agricultural entrepreneurship is:

- To stabilise market prices of agricultural commodities
- To get assured income from farm produce

- To generate additional income by utilizing farm produce
- To utilize the additional revenue or surplus money for the profitable business
- To generate income to sustain a family
- To achieve sustainable and equitable development

2. Twin role of the university in creating agricultural entrepreneurship

There are two basic approaches for universities/research institutions to create entrepreneurship. One approach is to commercialize the technology created (knowledge and materials) to generate revenue as a means of recovering technology development costs as well as providing financial support for their sustenance. universities or research institutions are setting up institutional arrangements such as technology transfer offices or units, incubators, technology information centres, etc., and seed funds to increase the commercialization of research. The Intellectual property is protected, which are then licensed to start-ups or other enterprises. This process is relatively new and many universities or research institutions are still learning to institutionalise them. The second approach is developing and creating expertise through entrepreneurial education for catalysing the entrepreneurial process. Several agricultural universities have introduced Business Management courses for creating a quality workforce to sustain the entrepreneurial activities.

For performing these roles the university provides technology support, mentoring and handholding support (Figure 1).

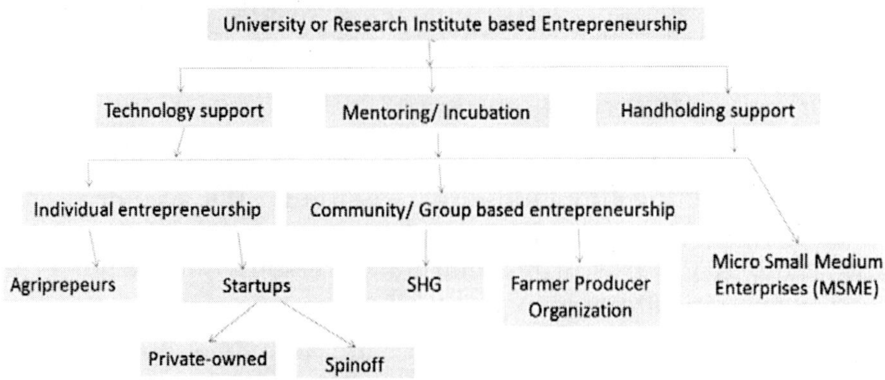

Figure 1: Role of university or research institute in entrepreneurship development

Types of agricultural entrepreneurs

A. Individual entrepreneurship

Agripreneurs

A new breed of entrepreneurs who combines their love of farming and agriculture with business. They can range from any age group; however, most are younger people getting back into the food business to bring healthy and better choices to the consumer.

Technology entrepreneur

A bold, imaginative deviator from established business methods and practices, who constantly seeks the opportunity to commercialize new products, technologies, processes, and arrangements. He/She is usually associated with start-ups.

Startups

Startups are baby companies, which are developing products or services based on a marketable idea, but yet to establish a concrete business model. They are basically upto five years from the date of its incorporation/registration, with an annual turnover - Maximum of ₹ 25 crore.

Micro Small Medium Enterprises

The MSMEs are classified into two types as given in Figure 2.

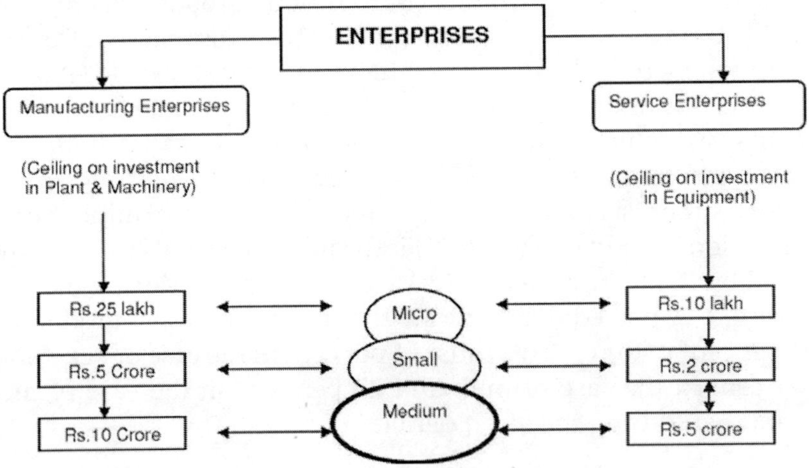

Figure 2: Classification of MSME

3. Importance of technology commercialisation in agriculture

Following facts indicate the need for commercialising agricultural technologies to maximise their impact on Indian society:

a) An instrument of poverty reduction

The agricultural commercialisation is promoted as an instrument for securing food security and reducing poverty. A World Bank study (Ravallion, and Datt, 1996) has estimated that a one per cent rise in agricultural value added per hectare results in a 0.4 per cent and 1.9 per cent reduction in poverty in the short- and long-run, respectively.

b) Rising share of high-value agriculture

Currently, India grows fruits and vegetables on less than 10 per cent of the area under all crops. CSO data on the value of output for the year 2013-14 reveals that fruits and vegetable crops on average generate ₹ 3.30 lakh worth of output per hectare compared with ₹ 37.5 thousand in the case of cereals and ₹ 29 thousand and ₹ 48.7 thousand in the cases of pulses and oilseeds, respectively (NITI Aayog, 2015). These variations in value productivity indicate a very large scope for raising the value of agricultural output through a shift from cereals, pulses and oilseeds into fruits and vegetables.

c) Shift in household dietary consumption patterns

The nature of eating and the composition of foods consumed has changed dramatically over the years. India's gross national income (per capita), increased by about 2.3 times in the last decade (2000-10), leaving surplus money in the hands of Indian consumers. Following Bennett's law, which states that sources of calories change with rising incomes, the cereal consumption has dramatically reduced in both rural and urban sectors in India. A recent National Sample Survey Organisation's study (NSSO, 2014) indicates that cereals consumption declined by 16.3% in rural and 12.4% in urban areas, during the 1993-2012 period. A pooled data indicate that per capita consumption rose by 21 per cent in the case of fruits, 14 per cent in the case of vegetables, 11 per cent in the case of milk and 23 per cent in the case of meat, eggs and fish during the same period.

d) Changes in the demographic composition of the Indian population

The age-related factors play a crucial role in agricultural commercialisation because of food consumption by individual changes over his/her lifetime. With 356 million 10-24 year-olds in 2011, India has the world's largest youth population. The rising youth brigade has the following implications (Swissnex India, 2015):

- **Entrepreneurial advantage** : The rising youth population has provided India with an advantage to harness the raw and energetic talent to create new start-ups on emerging technologies. However, the number of local entrepreneurs growing every year in India is very low. The Globel Innovation Index 2014 ranks India at 76 out of 143 countries. Realising the need to harness youth energy, National Policy for Skill Development and Entrepreneurship 2015 is formulated and several programmes were initiated to equip the critical knowledge and skills among youth for developing their entrepreneurial attitude and skills (Ministry of Skill Development and Entrepreneurship, 2015).
- **Diversity of foods consumed** : The youth prefer a wide dietary diversity which provides an opportunity for the food service entrepreneurs to create innovative start-ups to cater to the youth needs. A 2013 survey by National Restaurant Association of India indicated that nearly 61% of adolescents (14-17 years of age) eat out once a week, which shows an increasing trend (National Restaurant Association of India, 2013). In 2013, the size of the Indian foodservice industry was estimated at ₹ 247,680 crore, which is projected to grow to ₹ 408,040 crore by 2018 at 11% annual growth rate trend (National Restaurant Association of India, 2013).

e) Growth in Export Opportunities for High-Value Agricultural Commodities

The trade liberalization and domestic market reforms in India during the 1990s have opened up opportunities for the export of high-value commodities. Trade in high-value products is increasingly displacing exports of traditional commodities, such as rice, sugar, tea, co-ffee, tobacco, *etc*. For example, in India, during the 2000s, the growth rate in the value of exports of rice, sugar, tea, *etc*. declined, while high-value exports (fruits and vegetables, flowers, red meat, processed fruit juices) grew by about 18 per cent annually (Sharma and Jain, 2011).

f) Emerging agri-food retail chains

The Indian retail industry has emerged as one of the most dynamic and fast-paced industries due to the entry of several new players. It accounts for over 10 per cent of the country's Gross Domestic Product (GDP) and around 8 per cent of the employment. The retail industry in India is expected to grow to US$ 1.3 trillion by 2020, registering a Compound Annual Growth Rate (CAGR) of 16.7 per cent over 2015-20 (BCG and RAI, 2015). Grocery and food account for more than 50 per cent of fast-moving consumer goods (FMCG) sales and together form the biggest retail channel in India. This retail revolution is not only transforming the way South Asian consumers buy their food but also dictating how food is produced, graded, stored and displayed. Strengthening agri-food supply chains is the key outcome of this food retail revolution and it creates a wide range of business opportunities along the supply chain.

g) Increase in the FDI inflow for agri-businesses

Foreign Direct Investment (FDI) has been shown to play an important role in promoting economic growth, raising a country's technological level, and creating new employment in developing countries. Globalisation has led to an inflow of FDI into Indian agribusinesses that focus on higher-value and processed products (Regmi and Dyck, 2001). The FDI in agriculture can be made in three sectors such as food processing, agricultural services and agricultural machinery. Food processing industry is a predominant segment in the Food Industry in India, which contributes 6.3 per cent of the Gross Domestic Product of India (12 per cent of agricultural GDP), 19 per cent to the Indian industry, and 13 per cent to the export production. The food processing is a hallmark sector attracting FDI at an increasing level. The FDI in food processing rose from ₹ 279.01 crore in 2007-08 to 3,982.88 in 2013-14 (MOFPI, 2015).

4. Mechanism of commercialising agricultural technologies

The technology commercialisation process at the university or research institute (Figure 3) begins with the inventor, disclosing the research results to the organisations and urging them to assess their commercial potential. The Technology Transfer cell of the research organisation assesses the technology commercial viability and identifies prospective users. The viable technologies are protected by patents/copyright/trademarks/trade secrets and other forms of Intellectual Property protection. Based on the market assessment, the potential users of the technology are identified. The willing users can buy a licence for utilizing the technologies to realise its economic/ social or cultural benefits. The technologies that are not disclosed, are further researched through consultancy, collaborative or contract research, which are then protected. Other forms like publications, networking, academic spinoff, startups, etc. are also taken up for non-disclosed technologies.

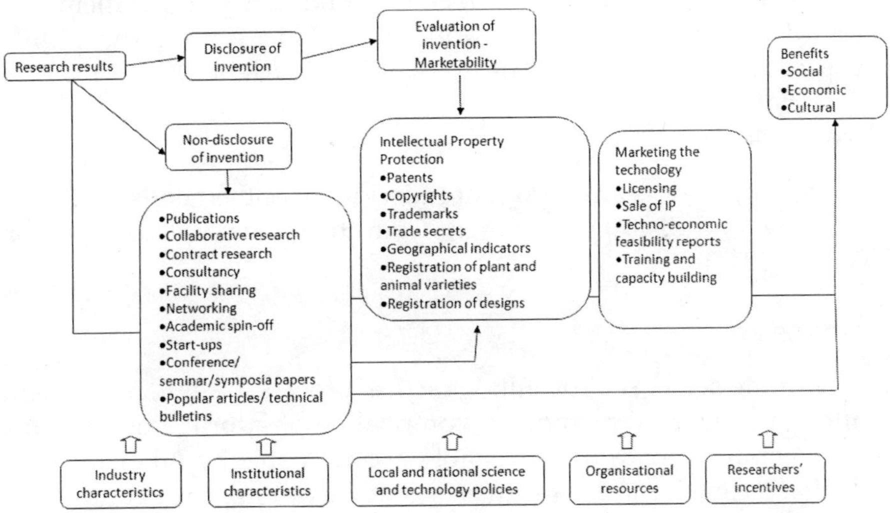

Figure 3: Technology commercialization process at ICAR-CTCRI

Means and modes of technology transfer

Intellectual property (IP)

The research results derived by its scientists/innovators in a research organisation or university, which could be protected by patents, plant variety protection or any other form of intellectual property rights, such as copyright, trademark, design, *etc.* This also includes know-how that may be protected as undisclosed information by suitable agreements.

Patent

A patent is a document, issued, upon application, by a government office (or a regional office acting for several countries), which describes an invention and creates a legal situation, in which the patented invention can normally only be exploited (manufactured, used, sold, imported) with the authorization of the owner of the patent (WIPO, 2008).

Copyright

Copyright is a right given by the law to creators of literary, dramatic, musical and artistic works and producers of cinematograph films and sound recordings. In fact, it is a bundle of rights including, *inter alia*, rights of reproduction, communication to the public, adaptation, and translation of the work (Copyright Office, 1999).

Trademark

A trademark is any sign that individualizes the goods of a given enterprise and distinguishes them from the goods of its competitors (WIPO, 2008).

Trade secret

A trade secret is a formula, practice, process, design, instrument, pattern, commercial method, or compilation of information, which is not generally known or reasonably ascertainable by others, and by which a business can obtain an economic advantage over competitors or customers (Lin, 2012).

Geographical indication

Geographical Indication is an indication that the good which is being commercialized under that indication has originated from a definite geographical territory either as agricultural produce (e.g. Nagpur orange) or natural produce, such as from mining (e.g. Mussourie Rock Phosphate) or by manufacturing (production or processing or preparation e.g. Banarasi saree) and it has a special quality or reputation or other characteristics attributable to that origin (ICAR, 2006).

Registration of plant or animal genetic resources or varieties

Registration of a plant variety gives protection only in India and confers upon the rights holder, its successor, agent, or licensee the exclusive right to produce, sell, market, distribute, import, or export the variety (Goel and Parashar, 2013).

Sponsored research

Where a university conceives a research project and prepare a proposal for funding and where the funding agency is not directly a beneficiary of the research results (Hamano, 2011).

Collaborative research

Research collaboration between a public university and private research unit of an enterprise or private organization (Hamano, 2011).

Contract research

Research collaboration between two entities, usually a research organisation or university and industry, for jointly developing technologies. This research is conceived and funded by industries/ government agencies to provide a solution to a specific problem (Hamano, 2011). The IP generated from the contract research is protected by the terms specified in the agreement.

Consultancy

A consultant contract is a legal agreement between a consultant and a client, by means of which the client buys the services of the consultant. The consultancy may involve providing expert advice and facilities for starting a technology-based enterprise, guidance in managing the enterprise profitably by solving the issues and problems, etc.

Spin-off

The spin-off is a separate company established in order to bring to the market technology developed by a public sector research organisation or university. The spin-offs are considered as a fundamental mediator between the research environment and industries, as they are a powerful means of technology transfer between these two sectors (European IPR Helpdesk, 2014). For example,

Agrinnovate (http://agrinnovateindia.co.in/) is a spin-off created by Indian Council of Agricultural Research (ICAR), India to commercialise its technologies.

Startup company

A startup company or startup is an entrepreneurial venture or a new business in the form of a company, a partnership or temporary organization designed to search for a repeatable and scalable business model.

Licensing

Licensing means the document embodying legal permission from a Research Organisation or University to the other party(is) to use its technologies/IP/Knowledge for commercial or other purposes under the terms and conditions and limitations, including a licence fee and/ or royalty, as negotiated and specified in the licence (ICAR, 2006).

Techno-economic feasibility report

This report outlines all the aspects which determine the feasibility of a technology-based enterprise. It provides a detailed description of the requirements for developing a technology-based industry including technology procurement, setting up the manufacturing facility, cost-benefit analysis, etc.

References

BCG-RAI, (2015). Retail 2020: retrospect, reinvent and rewrite. Leadership perspectives on trends in Indian retail. Retail Leadership Summit. Available at: http://www.bcgindia.com/documents/file181823.pdf

Copyright Office, (1999). A hand book of copyright law. Copyright Office, Ministry of Human Resource Development, Govt of India. Available at: http://copyright.gov.in/documents/handbook.html

European IPR Helpdesk, (2015). Fact Sheet Commercialising Intellectual Property: Spin-offs. The European IPT Helpdesk. Available at: https://www.iprhelpdesk.eu/sites/default/files/newsdocuments/Fact-Sheet-Commercializing-IP-Spin-offs.pdf

Goel, D., and Parashar, S. (2013). *IPR, Biosafety and Bioethics*. Noida, India: Dorling Kindersley (India) Pvt. Ltd.

Hamano, Y. (2011). Commercialization Procedures: Licensing, Spinoffs and Start-ups. World Intellectual Property Organisation. Available at: http://www.wipo.int/edocs/mdocs/aspac/en/wipo_ip_han_11/wipo_ip_han_11_ref_t7b.pdf

ICAR (2006). ICAR *Guidelines for Intellectual Property Management and Technology Transfer/ Commercialization*. New Delhi, Indian Council of Agriculture Research.

Lin, T.C.W. (2012). Executive Trade Secrets (April 28, 2012). 87 Notre Dame Law Review 911. Available at SSRN: http://ssrn.com/abstract=2047462

Ministry of Finance, (2011). Economic Survey 2010-11. Govt. of India.

Ministry of Skill Development and Entrepreneurship, (2015). Background. Available at: http://www.skilldevelopment.gov.in/background.html

National Restaurant Association of India, (2013). India Food Service Report 2013. National Restaurant Association of India. Available at: http://nrai.org/downloads/reports/

NITI Aayog, (2015). Raising Agricultural Productivity and Making Farming Remunerative for Farmers - An occasional paper. NITI Aayog Government of India. Available at: http://niti.gov.in/mgov_file/Raising%20Agricultural%20Productivity%20and%20Making% 20Farming%20Remunerative%20for%20Farmers.pdf

NSSO, (2014). *Nutritional Intake in India, 2011-12. NSS 68th Round. (July 2011 - June 2012).* National Sample Survey Organisation, Ministry of Statistics and Programme Implementation, Govt of India.

Ravallion M., and Datt G. (1996) How important to India's poor is the sectoral composition of economic growth?. *World Bank Economic Review* 10: 1–25.

Sharma, V.P. and Dinesh J. (2011). *High-Value Agriculture in India: Past Trends and Future Prospects.* Working Paper#2011-07-02. Ahmedabad, India: Indian Institute of Management Regmi, A. and J. Dyck (2001) *Effects of urbanization on global food demand. In: Changing Structures of Global Food Consumption and Trade*, edited by Anita Regmi. ERS WRS 01-1., USDA, ERS, Washington DC.

swissnex India, (2015). Social entrepreneurship in India - Unveiling the unlimited opportunities. Bangalore, swissnex India l Consulate General of Switzerland. Available at: http:// www. swissnexindia.org

WIPO, (2008). WIPO Intellectual Property Handbook: Policy, Law and Use. World Intellectual Property Organisation. Available at: http://www.wipo.int/edocs/pubdocs/en/intproperty/489/wipo_pub_489.pdf

Chapter 20

Patent Search by Using Different Databases

R. Selvam

The "Patent Search" is a method of examining for the documents that will determine whether an invention is novel and non-obvious and it may meet the requirements for granting a patent or not? Patent searches usually originate with a database of issued patents, patent applications and also include other types of documents, such as journal articles and scientific papers that describe unpatented inventions. A patent search can be done by the inventor itself or hiring a patent search professionals, namely a patent agent or patent attorney or private searcher.

Purpose of a Patent Search

- A researcher would like to list out the patents in a certain field, which helps in guiding his research, identify specific new ideas and technical solutions, products or processes and for improvement of an existing product or process (Prior art / State-of-the-Art search).
- An inventor would like to make sure that his invention is unique before he spends time and money to obtain a patent (Patentability/Novelty search).
- An organization would like to produce a product and wants to make sure that they do not get sued by someone else that might have already patented that idea (Freedom to operate search / Infringement search).
- An organization is making a product and is being sued by another organization, which believes it holds a patent on that product, and the first organization would like to prove that the second organization's patent is invalid (Validity search).

Types of patent searches

The patent searches conducted for a different purpose and has a different approach.

	Prior art search	Patentability	Validity Search	Infringement Search	Freedom to operate search
Description	Previously used or published technology that may be referred to in a patent.	Patentability/ Novelty search is typically performed before filing a patent in order to determine whether or not the invention is novel and non-obvious.	A search conducted with the intent of finding prior art to invalidate a pre-existing patent.	A search conducted for the purpose of determining, if a given product or process would infringe upon any in-force patent claims	Searching the claims of third-party in-force patents to determine, if the claims of any prior art read on aspects of the technology that is to enter the market place.
Coverage	Worldwide Patents and Applications	Worldwide Patents and Applications and Non-Patent literature. Any product/technical presentation	Worldwide Patents and Applications and Non-Patent literature. Any product/technical presentation	Worldwide Patents and Applications	Active patents of a particular country where the product under question is to be manufactured
Date Range	All	All	Documents dated till the critical date of the query patent	Active patents	Active patents and expired patents (if required)
Area of focus in patent	The query in Full text of the documents	The query in Full text of the documents	The claim of the query patent in full text of the documents	The claim of the query patent in claims of other patents	The query in claims of the patents
Result	List of issued patents and published application	List of issued patents, published application, non-patent literature, and patentability opinion	List of issued patents, published application, non-patent literature and Validity opinion	List of issued patents and Infringement opinion	List of issued patents and Freedom to operate opinion

Other patent searches are viz.

a) Patent Family Search

This kind of search is carried out to identify a member of a "patent family." Patent family searches are used to find the countries, in which a given patent application has been filed and to obtain a list of references cited and to estimate the importance of the invention (by a number of patent documents relating to the same invention and being published in different countries).

b) Cited or Citing References Search

A patent may refer to or be referenced by important documents that may be crucial for making an improvement to an existing invention. Cited or Citing References search gives a comprehensive list of document that refers to a patent and documents that the patent refers to.

c) Inventor, Author or Assignee Search

Inventor, author or assignee search provides a complete list of document that belongs to a particular inventor, author or assignee.

Patent search process

The various ways of searching patent databases are as follows:

Hand Search

This is basically a patent by patent manual search. The patents are filed by classes and subclasses. This type of search is conducted in the public search room at the patent office.

Computer Search

This is basically a searching patent by using the online databases. Many national patent offices have launched free of charge patent information databases, which are open to the public. For example, the full text and full page image database of the United States Patent and Trademark Office (USPTO) is one of the earliest and free online patent information services. Another major online free patent database is espacenet, which has some 30 million patent documents. There are a number of private companies that have commercial databases. These include Derwent, Dialog, STN, Questel Orbit, Micropatent, Delphion, etc. Commercial services offer enhanced or value-added patent information, based on the actual requirement of particular end-users.

Literature Search

This is a search of the published literature to locate patents. This can be easily done in a library that has the abstract volumes of the particular science concerned. Chemical Abstracts, Electronic Abstracts, Physical Abstracts, etc., are typical sources of data.

Important databases for patent search

Patent Offices

- The United States Patent and Trademark Office, (http://patft.uspto.gov)
- European Patent Office (http://ep.espacenet.com)
- World Intellectual Property Organization (www.wipo.int)
- Indian Patent Office (http://ipindia.nic.in/patsea.htm)
- Non-Patent Literature
- Pubmed (www.ncbi.nlm.nih.gov/sites/entrez)
- Science Direct (www.sciencedirect.com)

Commercial database

- Delphion (www.delphion.com)
- Micro-Patent (www.micropatent.com)
- The STN (www.cas.org)
- Genome Quest (www.genomequest.com)

Others

- Google Patents (www.google.com/patents)
- Free Patents Online (www.freepatentsonline.com)
- Patent Lens (www.patentlens.net)
- India Big patents (http://india.bigpatents.org)

Patent search tools

There are different tools used in conducting the patent search are as given below:

A. Keyword Search

A keyword search is querying a patent database, using the keywords. A process of carrying out a keyword search is by identifying words that define the features of the invention, identify synonymous for the keywords and form key strings that can be used as a search query in the database. The search may also specify the fields or parts of patents. Keyword searches are quick and suitable for very recently developed technology for which patent classifications are not yet developed. The inventors may not have used the same words for describing an invention in the patents. So, it is crucial to develop a good list of keywords and it's synonymous, and then implement the searches with appropriate logic.

Boolean Operators

Boolean operators help to combine words or phrases to broaden or narrow the search. Boolean operators can be used to specify what we want and what we do not want while searching.

Boolean Operator	Example	Function
AND	Drug and Formulation	Finds documents, which have both drug and formulation.
OR	Drug or Formulation	Finds documents, which have either drug or formulation or both.
NOT	Drug not Formulation	Finds documents, which have the only drug.

Nested Queries/Creating queries with Parentheses or Brackets

The search terms and its Boolean operators can be enclosed in parentheses or brackets to specify the order in which they should be processed. Information within parentheses is read first and then information outside parentheses.

Nested query	How it is interpreted
Hair and dye or colourant	Hair and (dye or colourant)

Wildcards

Wildcard or truncation search used to retrieve documents containing variations of a search term. Wildcard symbols can be used to replace a single letter or a part of a word, or one or more numbers.

Query	Results list would have
Standardification	Standardisation and Standardization
Col*r	Colour and Colour

The wildcard for USPTO is "$" and for Delphion, Espacenet, WIPO databases is "*".

Proximity Search

Proximity search helps to specify how near/distant the search terms must be. The distance or nearness of the terms searched can be specified as whole numbers. The proximity operator is "~". The proximity operator should be followed by a whole number indicating the proximity of the search terms.

Query	Results list would have
"Mastitis Treatment"~5	Documents with both mastitis and treatment and within five words of each other.

Word Stemming

Word stemming is a language related tool, which determines the root of a word first, and then retrieves all possible variants. If word stemming ON, documents with both the root word and its variants will be retrieved and if word stemming OFF, the search is limited to the exact word.

Term	Word Stemming	Matching results would have the word(s)
Composition	Off (searches for the exact word)	Composition
Composition	On (searches for variants of the root word "compose")	Composition, Compositions, Compose, compose, composed, composing, etc.

Search Term Weighting

The "^" (caret) operator is used for search term weighting. The caret "^" should be followed by a whole number that indicates relative importance.

Query	Interpretation
Catalyst^5 or Reagent	The catalyst is 5 times more important than Reagent. Finds all documents with either Catalyst or Reagent, or both, rank documents with Catalyst higher.

B. Classification Search

Patent classification is a way by which the documents, such as patent applications, disclosing inventions are arranged according to the technical features of inventions. Each patent application will be assigned one or more class based on the technology to which it relates. The patent offices assign classes to the patent applications. Hence, by using patent classification codes as search query, patent documents filed across various patent offices can be searched.

There are various classification systems. The International Patent Classification (IPC) is agreed internationally. The United States Patent Classification (USPC) is by the United States Patent and Trademark Office. The European Classification (ECLA) is based on the IPC but adapted by the European Patent Office. The Derwent classification system is fixed by an enterprise. Since classification searching relies on the features of a patent, rather than the words used to describe the patent, all patents that utilize specific features will be returned as a search result.

C. Patent Number Search

The patent numbers are displayed in products or packaging or available in the "non-patent" literature, such as scientific and technical reports can be used to search the concerned patents.

D. Date Range Search

Patent documents bear several dates (date of application, priority date, and date of grant). These dates are very important to decide the age of an invention and to the question of whether the inventions they describe are still under legal protection. If they are no longer legally protected, they can be used without the consent of the patentee.

Date range searching is searching patents, which are filed or published during a defined period of time. For example, the search query, "APD/10/22/1986->10/21/2006 and recombinant and vaccine" will retrieve all patents applied for between October 22, 1986, and October 21, 2006, that contain the words recombinant and vaccine.

Value of patent search results

The patent search helps the inventor in decision making. The patent search can save the inventor's time and money spent on an idea that is not original. The patent search needs to be done to find all similar patents and then draft the patent application accordingly. A complete report will show what areas of the idea need to change, if they conflict with existing patents or which areas of the idea to be further developed, as they are truly original. If the invention is found to be original through the patent search, the results will help the wording of the patent application, so it is more likely to be granted. The patent search results will always be useful either if the invention was found to be original or not and it helps to decide what to do next.